THE OLDER P

An Introduction to Ge

CW00485860

MODERN NURSING SERIES

General Editor
SUSAN E. NORMAN SRN, DNCert, RNT
Senior Tutor, The Nightingale School, St. Thomas's Hospital, London

Consultant Editor

A. J. HARDING RAINS MS, FRCS
Regional Dean, British Postgraduate Medical Federation
Formerly Professor of Surgery, Charing Cross Hospital Medical School
Honorary Consultant Surgeon, Charing Cross Hospital
Honorary Consultant Surgeon to the Army

This series caters for the needs of a wide range of nursing, medical and ancillary professions. Some of the titles are given below, but a complete list is available from the Publisher.

Gerontology and Geriatric Nursing
SIR W. FERGUSON ANDERSON OBE, KStJ, MD, FRCP
F. I. CAIRD MA, DM, FRCP
R. D. KENNEDY MB, ChB, FRCP
D. SCHWARTZ BS, MA, RN

Textbook of Medicine
R. J. HARRISON ChB, MD

Principles of Medicine and Medical Nursing
J. C. HOUSTON CBE, MD, FRCP
H. HYDE WHITE SRN

Surgery and Surgical Nursing
S. TAYLOR DM, MCh, FRCS, HonFRCS (Ed), HonFCS (SA)
M. BIRCHALL SRN, RCNT

Revision Notes on Psychiatry
K. T. KOSHY MSc, SRN, BTA, RMN, RNT, ARIPHH, MRSH

Community Health and Social Services
J. B. MEREDITH DAVIES MD, FFCM, DPH

Other relevant titles:
The 36-Hour Day
N. MACE, P. V. RABINS, B. CASTLETON, C. CLOKE, E. McEWEN

Learning to Care for Elderly People
L. THOMAS

THE OLDER PATIENT

An Introduction to Geriatric Nursing

Fourth Edition

R. E. Irvine

CBE, MA, MD, FRCP
Consultant Physician
Department of Medicine for the Elderly
Hastings Health Authority

M. K. Bagnall

AIMSW
Independent Social Work Consultant
Formerly Principal Hospital Social Worker
Social Services Department, East Sussex County Council

B. J. Smith

SRN, RFN
Formerly Area Nursing Officer, Doncaster
and Matron, St. Helen's and Royal East Sussex Hospitals, Hastings

with the assistance of

V. A. Bishop

SRN, ONC, RCNT
St Wilfrid's Hospice, Eastbourne
Formerly Clinical Teacher, ENB Course, The Care of the Elderly
Hastings School of Nursing

HODDER AND STOUGHTON
LONDON SYDNEY AUCKLAND TORONTO

Dedication

To all those who have cared for our patients in and out of hospital.
They have taught us more than they know.

Irvine, R. E.
  The older patient: an introduction to geriatric
  nursing.—4th ed.—(Modern nursing series)
  1. Geriatrics   2. Geriatric nursing
  I. Title   II. Bagnall, M. K.   III. Smith, B. J.
  (Barbara Janet)   IV. Series
  618.97'0024613   RC952

ISBN 0 340 37682 1

First published 1968
Second edition 1970
Third impression 1976
Third edition 1978
Second impression 1983
Fourth edition 1986

Typeset in 11/12 pt Bembo by Macmillan India Ltd., Bangalore 25.

Printed in Great Britain for
Hodder and Stoughton Educational,
a division of Hodder and Stoughton Limited,
Mill Road, Dunton Green, Sevenoaks, Kent
Printed in Great Britain by
Richard Clay (The Chaucer Press) Ltd,
Bungay, Suffolk

Editors' Foreword

This well established series of books reflects contemporary nursing and health care practice. It is used by a wide range of nursing, medical and ancillary professions and encompasses titles suitable for different levels of experience from those in training to those who have qualified.

Members of the nursing professions need to be highly informed and to keep critically abreast of demanding changes in attitudes and technology. The series therefore continues to grow with new titles being added to the list and existing titles being updated regularly. Its aim is to promote sound understanding by presenting essential facts clearly and concisely. We hope this will lead to nursing care of the highest standard.

Foreword to the First Edition

With over half the patients in most medical and orthopaedic wards over the age of sixty, and a large proportion of the patient-population of psychiatric hospitals also in this age category, it can be said with some truth that geriatric nursing today is more of a generality than a speciality. The mere presence of elderly patients, however, does not automatically sponsor enlightenment of their special needs. In the growing awareness of this, progressive Geriatric Departments are finding themselves increasingly regarded as sources of information and as centres of education on the complexities of the care and welfare of the older patient. The appearance of this book, therefore, is particularly timely.

It is all the more valuable in that it embodies the combined experience of a doctor, a nurse, and a medical social worker, thereby demonstrating the first essential for the successful practice of geriatrics, namely, that it is wholly dependent upon teamwork.

From its pages the nurse will not only gain insight into his or her role in the team, but also, with subsequent practical experience, discover two ungarnished truths. Firstly, far from being dull, geriatric nursing holds exciting opportunities for pitting wits and skill against real practical nursing problems. Secondly, having learnt to nurse old people successfully in all the phases of acute illness, rehabilitation and long-term care, one is then equipped to nurse anybody, with any condition, anywhere.

Doreen Norton

Foreword to the Fourth Edition

As one of a generation of nurses who undertook training without the benefit of experience in geriatric nursing, *The Older Patient* was my first introduction to the exciting opportunities of the specialty promised by Doreen Norton in her foreword to the first edition.

In the intervening years, there have been many changes and fresh challenges. Nursing itself has developed a more systematic approach to planning care, while growing emphasis on care in the community has led to a better understanding of the vital role which families and other carers play in supporting old people at home.

These and other changes are reflected in this radically revised fourth edition. Some factors, however, have remained constant and none more so than the fundamental belief in a team approach to the care of elderly people.

As a raw recruit to the specialty all those years ago, this book not only provided me with a sound basis of knowledge on which to build, but also helped to open my mind.

A new generation of readers will continue to need imagination and ingenuity if the challenges of the future are to be dealt with effectively. I can think of no better place for them to start than within these pages.

Linda Thomas
Nurse Adviser
RCN Society of Geriatric Nursing

Preface to the Fourth Edition

Since our last edition appeared in 1978 the Health Service has been reorganised yet again and further changes are in store as new General Managers are appointed.

For the older patient, as for all other consumers of NHS resources, the problem has been how to give better care to more people without any matching increase in resources. This has led to increasing emphasis on care in the community. The expertise of the Primary Health Care Team and the domiciliary social services has improved. This has led to shorter stays in hospital for old people and an increasing emphasis in Departments of Geriatric Medicine on acute intervention. The best way to help an old person when he becomes ill is to get him into hospital quickly so that he may go home sooner with less risk of ending up as a long stay patient. This does not of course diminish the importance of high standards when long stay care in hospital or a nursing home is the best answer to the patient's problem.

In reality community care means more care for old people by their relatives. Better ways of helping caring families are being developed and the carers themselves have found a voice through the new Association of Carers.

The elderly now outnumber the children in our schools and their importance as consumers is being increasingly recognised. Organisations like Age Concern, Help the Aged and the Centre for Policy on Ageing have done much to create public awareness and to alert society to the problems of the elderly. To have such powerful advocates has done much to raise morale among the elderly.

Finally the private sector is increasing. Since the Supplementary Benefit Regulations were changed in 1982 it has been possible for many elderly people who could not previously have afforded it to receive care in the private sector. This arrangement widens the older patient's opportunities for choice and has greatly helped the hospital geriatric service by making discharge easier.

In previous editions of this book there was a section describing the illnesses of the older patient. This has now been deleted to make room for a more extended consideration of nursing matters.

There are now numerous excellent books on geriatric medicine from Professor J. C. Brocklehurst's great textbook of *Geriatric Medicine and Gerontology* (Churchill Livingstone) to shorter summaries such as Professor H. M. Hodkinson's *Outline of Geriatrics* (Academic Press) and Genet Adam's *Essentials of Geriatric Medicine* (Oxford University Press). *Geriatrics* by A. N. Exton-Smith and P. W. Overstall (MTP Press), *Geriatric Medicine* by R. C. Hamdy (Pitman) and *Lecture Notes on Geriatrics* by N. Coni, W. Davison and S. Webster (Blackwell) are also strongly recommended.

There are now so many books on gerontology and geriatrics that we have made recommendations for further reading at the end of each chapter.

We hope that a new generation of readers will find these changes acceptable.

R. E. Irvine
M. K. Bagnall
B. J. Smith
V. A. Bishop

Acknowledgments

It is a pleasure to acknowledge the continued help and support which we have enjoyed from the Hastings Health Authority, the District Management Team and from our colleagues in every discipline. We are particularly grateful to Theodore Strouthidis, Pamela Kendall and the staff of the Department of Medicine for the Elderly, to Tom Venkateswarlu and his team in the Department of Mental Health for the Elderly and to our surgical colleagues, Michael Devas, Barry Hinves, Charles Gallannaugh, John Shepperd and David Rees, with whom we have worked closely over many years.

Our nursing colleagues have laboured to maintain standards under difficult circumstances and we continue to be grateful to Marjorie Couchman, Ben Williams, Sandy Ward, Kathleen Davies, Margaret Earland and many others. We are particularly grateful also to those students and teachers who have contributed to our lively ENB courses in the Care of the Elderly. It is a pleasure also to record our debt to the physiotherapists and occupational therapists who continue to be directed by Eleanor Chambers and Pat Hunter. We are grateful also to our speech therapist, Sue Caroll, for her valuable help at all times but also for her fine example in starting the Hastings District's first stroke club.

Once again we are indebted to Norma Waterman for her illustrations and to Marjorie Roscoe, Joan Burt, Beth Hodge and Dawn Noakes, who have most kindly and patiently offered secretarial help.

Sources of Information

Information about furniture and equipment, the indispensable tools for the care of the older patient, is available from the Kings Fund Centre, 126 Albert Street, London NW1 2 NF. The staff of the Centre can put enquirers in touch with the appropriate manufacturers. The monthly publication, *Hospital Equipment and Supplies*, provides an up-to-date view of current ideas in furniture and equipment. For general reference the catalogues of the major hospital suppliers are invaluable.

The main source of information about all kinds of aids is The Disabled Living Foundation, 380—4 Harrow Road, London W9 2HU (tel. 01 289 6111). The Foundation publishes regular information sheets and maintains an Aids Centre where a wide range of equipment and special clothing is available for demonstration.

New ideas and comment appear frequently in the nursing journals to which the *British Journal of Geriatric Nursing* is a most important recent addition.

Physiotherapy and the *British Journal of Occupational Therapy* continue to provide a great deal of information about the elderly and *Therapy* is a weekly newspaper for the remedial professions. *Social Work Today* and *Community Care* are two social work journals which are always worth reading. *Ageing and Society* provides a forum for research papers in social gerontology.

Specialist medical publications include *Age and Ageing*, the journal of the British Geriatrics Society and the British Society for Research on Ageing, Gerontology and Geriatric Medicine, which is aimed at general practitioners.

Baseline, the journal of the British Association for Service to the Elderly (Base), is a multidisciplinary publication of wide interest.

Consumer orientated journals include *Choice*, the magazine of the Pre-retirement Association (PRA). It emphasises the many opportunities now open to retired people. *New Age*, the journal of Age Concern, and *Yours*, published by Help the Aged, both give opportunities for the elderly themselves, as well as those who help them, to express their views.

Contents

The older patient and his further nursing needs

Quality of care

Introduction

Geriatrics

Geriatrics is the branch of medicine which deals with the diseases and problems of old age. Because much of the illness to which old people are prone tends to run a prolonged course, geriatrics is associated in many people's minds with 'chronic sickness', an unfortunate term giving a wholly misleading picture of what goes on in a modern Department of Geriatric Medicine. As anyone who works in such a department will discover, the greater part of the work is concerned with the older patient in acute illness, with his rehabilitation and with his ultimate return to the community. Only a small proportion, less than one in ten, of the patients who come to a Department of Geriatric Medicine require prolonged nursing care. This too has its own challenges and rewards.

Population changes

Geriatrics has emerged as a new specialty in medicine and nursing because there has been a phenomenal increase in the numbers of elderly all over the world. Two-thirds of all those who have ever reached the age of 65 in the history of the world are alive at the present time.

In England and Wales, at the beginning of the present century, the total population was 30 million. Only 5 per cent were over 65 and there were less than half a million people over 75. Today the population is just over 54 million of whom 8 million, almost 15 per cent, are over 65. There are now more than 3 million people over 75 accounting for 5.7 per cent or 1 in 17 of the population. During the next twenty years the total number of people over 65 will not increase, but within this total there will be a much greater proportion of the very old. Those between 65 and 74 were most numerous in 1978. Those between 75 and 84 will reach their peak in 1991. Those over 85 will reach their greatest numbers in the year 2001, their numbers having increased by 60 per cent since 1978.

These figures represent averages for the country as a whole. In retirement areas like the South Coast more than a quarter of the population may be elderly. In industrial areas the proportion of the elderly is less.

Old age is largely a woman's world. Over 75 there are twice as many women as men and over 85 four times as many. Two-thirds of the women are widows (only one in six over 85 still has a husband). These are the people who make the greatest demands on the medical and social services. On any one day half of all the hospital beds in the country are occupied by people over 65.

In 1980 there were 185,000 people resident in homes run by local authorities, voluntary organisations or privately. It is important to remember, however, that 95 per cent of old people still live in private households. Similar patterns are apparent in Europe, Russia and North America.

Pattern of disease

All this is due to the greatly improved expectation of life brought about by improved economic conditions, higher standards of living and modern medicine. Since 1900 the average expectation of life has increased by more than 20 years. In Britain men now have an expectation of life at birth of 70 and women of 76. In Sweden and Japan the expectation of life at birth is even higher, 73 for men and 78 for women. Formerly many people died in childhood or early adult life from infectious diseases such as pneumonia, typhoid, tuberculosis and diphtheria, all of which can now be prevented or cured.

The people who would have died of these diseases in the past now live on to old age, so that one in five women and one in ten men can expect to live to the age of 85. As they grow older they are more likely to develop one or more of the illnesses common in old age, for example arthritis, stroke or mental illness. These and many other diseases to which the older patient is vulnerable may cause prolonged disability. In England three-quarters of a million elderly people, the majority of them over 75, have severe physical and mental handicaps. The management of these patients is the main challenge of geriatric medicine.

At present very little is known about the prevention of disease in old age. It is important not to smoke, to be moderate in eating and drinking, to take as much exercise as possible and to make every effort to remain interested in life. Once people have reached the age of 65 their further expectation of life has increased by only one and a half years for men and four years for women in the past hundred years. Nevertheless a woman reaching 70 today has, as she did then, a further expectation of life of twelve years and a man nine years. At 80 she can expect another seven years and he another five.

Change in hospital

Because old people are more prone to disease than younger ones, and because the proportion of old people in the population is steadily growing, a typical general hospital ward, medical, surgical, orthopaedic or psychiatric, will have at least half of its beds filled with patients of pensionable age and the proportion is steadily increasing.

Understanding of the problems of the elderly is improving but at the same time it has become apparent that the more difficult problems of the older patient are easier to solve in an environment where special skills and experience, both clinical and social, are available. For these reasons geriatric nursing, like geriatric medicine, has emerged as a specialty. In 1962 the General Nursing Council included geriatrics among the subjects for student nurse training, and in 1973 post-registration courses in the care of the elderly were set up by the Joint Board of Clinical Nursing Studies, and now the English National Board (ENB). We hope that this book will be helpful to nurses at all stages of their training as well as those in other disciplines whose work brings them into contact with the older patient.

Work with the elderly is full of interest. No field of patient care makes greater demands on human sympathy, energy and expertise. The needs of the elderly are so many and so various that no one profession can meet them alone. The nurse, the doctor, the remedial therapist, the social worker and many others bring their skills to the service of the patient and his family. None of them can be effective in isolation. The whole team is needed, and multidisciplinary team work is more highly developed in the medicine of the elderly than in any other field. The nurse who is clever enough or fortunate enough to become a member of such a team will find that work with the elderly is immensely rewarding.

For further reading:

CARVER, V & LIDDIARD, P (Eds). 1978. *An Ageing Population*. Sevenoaks: Hodder and Stoughton.
SHEGOG, R F A (Ed). 1981. *The Impending Crisis of Old Age*. Oxford: Oxford University Press.

I

Psychological Ageing

Old age is not entirely a matter of years. Some people remain young in their eighties while others seem old in their sixties. Eight out of ten people in the age group 65—74 enjoy good health but after 75 only 10 per cent are free of all health problems. One in three over 75 has difficulty in taking a bath, one in four some problems in getting around, but the majority find life worth living. In hospital the staff see only those who are ill. It is easy to forget that there are many more people, as old as the patients, living happy and fulfilled lives at home.

For the purpose of this book we shall regard the older patient as one who, if taken ill, would feel at home in a geriatric ward. In practice most patients in this category will be over 75 and one characteristic which they almost all have in common is a measure of dependence on others in their daily lives. They are changing from being contributors to the community to becoming the recipients of services from others.

In most official documents and statistics the elderly are considered to be all those who qualify for the Retirement Pension. In Great Britain this means women over 60 years and men over 65. However those in the early years of retirement are not usually troubled by the problems of old age. Most are able to maintain a fully independent life. But somewhere in the middle seventies a gradual change becomes apparent, perhaps occasioned by a fall or an illness. Old people cease to be fully independent and need an increasing amount of help from relatives, friends or the social services.

The process of ageing

The changes which mark this transition from the early to the later phases of senescence, are the culmination of a gradual process of ageing which has been going on quietly for about fifty years, beginning when the patient reached the peak of his development in his twenties or even earlier.

Growing old is a normal part of the cycle of human existence. Although old people are more prone to disease than younger ones, old age is not in itself a disease. It is, therefore, a great mistake to attribute all the troubles of the elderly to 'senility' which implies that nothing can be done about them. The illnesses of the elderly require to be investigated and treated with the same care and thoroughness as those of younger people, and their response to treatment is often very good.

The study of the ageing process is known as gerontology. This is now being pursued increasingly all over the world, especially in Russia, the United States, France and Britain. Gerontology is not a purely medical activity. It concerns biologists, psychologists and sociologists as well as doctors and nurses.

Ageing and mental processes

The mental changes associated with ageing are in many ways more important and sometimes more disabling than the physical. It is very hard sometimes to draw the line between what is normal for old age and what is pathological. Many of the difficulties involved in the care of the elderly spring from this cause.

Intelligence has many facets. Memory, comprehension, problem solving and speed of response can all be tested. So can the use of words, figures, shapes and pictures. Although most people show a decline with age in some tests of intelligence, there are many individual exceptions. It is only after the age of 80 that everyone shows some loss. But even in advanced age there are old people who do as well in some tests of intelligence as those who are much younger.

Slowing up

The older patient is likely to think and move more slowly than when he was young. He is a creature of habit. He distrusts new experiences and prefers the old and familiar. He is in no hurry to make decisions and when faced with a new problem takes longer to solve it. A capacity to tackle new situations depends on what is called fluid intelligence which declines with age. But this does not mean that the saying 'you can't teach an old dog new tricks' is wholly true. The older patient can learn new things but he needs time. He cannot be hurried, a point which the nurse, who is inevitably in a hurry, must try to remember.

There is another kind of intelligence called crystallised intelligence, consisting of all the information the older patient has acquired throughout life. It enables him to use familiar words and numbers without deterioration and is the basis of the wisdom of old age.

Memory

Some loss of memory, especially for recent events, is almost universal in old age. At first it may be no more than a difficulty in recalling names and dates, but later an old person may be unable to remember who came to see him and what happened yesterday. Eventually he may become very absent-minded and forget where he put his spectacles five minutes ago.

Recent memory is much more impaired in old age than is memory of the distant past. Old people whose memories are beginning to fail sometimes surprise their visitors by the vividness with which they can recall their childhood perhaps seventy years before. This unfortunately is a mixed blessing since it may lead to a tendency to live in the past and to be unrealistic about the present. Impairment of recent memory may make it hard for old people to give an accurate account of their illness or social circumstances, and this must be taken into account by those who try to help them. One should never presume to discount or ignore what an old person says, but it is desirable to check the information whenever possible. An old person may also find it hard to remember future plans and may need to be reminded of these repeatedly.

Emotional changes

The emotional needs of people at any age are the same. We all need affection, to feel wanted and to be of use to others. At the same time we need to feel independent, and to have the sense of security which comes from sufficient food, warmth and shelter. In old age it is harder to satisfy these needs. Many old people become isolated, and the oldest are likely to have outlived family and friends. They may thus find themselves increasingly lonely at an age when new friendships and social contacts are difficult to establish.

Some old people seem to become blunted in their emotions and show no strong feelings of joy or sorrow, but there is a wide variety. One old person may accept the loss of a lifelong partner with remarkable equanimity. Another may grieve as intensely as he would have done in earlier life. It is wise and humane for those who work with the elderly to assume that the patient feels things as acutely as they would were they in his shoes. Do as you would be done by is the golden rule.

Old people tire easily as their physical and mental powers wane. Some can accept their infirmities philosophically, but others become apprehensive and sense a threat to their security from the increasing restrictions of their lives. This situation is often aggravated by financial hardship. Others again may become depressed at the deprivations of old age and may react by apathy, withdrawal and self-neglect. Suicide is commoner in old age than at any other time of life, especially amongst men.

Sex

Interest in the opposite sex remains throughout life and is natural and wholesome. Old people in hospital and residential homes, though generally preferring single sex bedrooms, benefit from mixed company by day. If a couple should become attached to one another, expressions of affection are normal and to be encouraged.

Sexual activity slowly declines throughout adult life, but even after the age of 75 one couple in four still enjoys sex and for those who no longer have intercourse, tenderness, affection and physical closeness are as valuable in old age as at any other time of life.

Sleep

In old age there are changes in the pattern of sleep which becomes more fragmented. Elderly people take longer to go to sleep. Their sleep is lighter and they waken more often. They are more likely to take naps during the day, but their night time sleep, seven to eight hours, is the same as in younger people. Throughout adult life women sleep differently from men, spending more time in bed and waking less often during the night.

A variety of sleep complaints occur in the elderly and these are reflected in their wide consumption of sleeping pills. The changes in sleep pattern which are part of normal ageing become more abnormal if the patient has organic brain disease.

Personality changes

Although the mental changes of old age may follow a fairly recognisable pattern, this does not prevent the old person from retaining his individual personality. Indeed, in old age there is often an apparent exaggeration of personal characteristics. The old person may become, it has been said, a caricature of his former self.

The adult learns to mask his true feelings in order to make himself socially acceptable; the old person tends to be less inhibited in his behaviour. He may find it harder to guard his tongue and to control his actions. Minor frustrations which he would once have shrugged off may provoke outbursts of temper and jealousy. He may become more self-centred, petty or suspicious. He may be increasingly close with money, not always from necessity, and some old people become hoarders. He may deteriorate in his personal habits, paying less attention to table manners, dress and personal hygiene.

The mental changes of old age are not always for the worse, however. Those who age most successfully manifest a serenity and detachment from the trials of daily life which is worthy of profound admiration. The following is an extract of a broadcast made by Mr J. W. Robertson Scott on his 91st birthday. It expresses perfectly the achievement of successful ageing.

'Do not be sorry for a man in his nineties as I am. He has three advantages. He has seen no end of forebodings of disaster come to nothing. He knows that the many changes that have taken place in his lifetime have been almost wholly for the better. He has undergone what I call the final discipline. By that I mean that he has usually come through what he may take to be the worst and the best that can happen to him.

'One gift that comes to the ageing is a relish for quiet, an appreciation of being alone. Another gain is a sense of proportion. The aged realise more and more fully what is important and what is less important, and what is not important at all.'

The importance of the individual

Whatever happens to him in old age, every person preserves his individuality as a human being and should therefore be treated as a person of consequence. One important way to do this is to address him by his proper name. To call an old person Dad or Gran or even Dear is to show that you are not sufficiently interested in him as an individual to remember his name. There is possibly no single lesson so important for those who work with the elderly as to realise that they are all individuals who just happen to be old.

The hunger of the old person to be recognised as an individual is memorably expressed in a poem by Mrs Phyllis McCormack, 'Look Closer', which appeared in the *Nursing Mirror* in 1972. It sums up this chapter admirably.

Look Closer

What do you see, nurse, what do you see?
Are you thinking when you are looking at me —
A crabbit old woman, not very wise
Uncertain of habit, with far-away eyes,
Who dribbles her food and makes no reply
When you say in a loud voice — 'I do wish you'd try'
Who seems not to notice the things that you do,
And forever is losing a stocking or shoe.
Who unresisting or not, lets you do as you will,
With bathing and feeding, the long day to fill,
Is that what you are thinking, is that when you see?
Then open your eyes, nurse, you're not looking at me.
I'll tell you who I am as I sit here so still;
As I use at your bidding, as I eat at your will,
I'm a small child of ten with a father and mother,
Brothers and sisters, who love one another.
A young girl of sixteen with wings on her feet,
Dreaming that soon now a lover she'll meet;
A bride soon at twenty — my heart gives a leap,
Remembering the vows that I promised to keep.
At twenty-five now I have young of my own,
Who need me to build a secure, happy home,
A woman of thirty, my young now grow fast,
Bound to each other with ties that should last;
At forty, my young sons have grown and are gone,
By my man's beside me to see I don't mourn;
At fifty, once more babies play round my knee,
Again we know children, my loved one and me.
Dark days are upon me, my husband is dead,
I look at the future, I shudder with dread,
For my young ones are all rearing young of their own,
And I think of the years and the love that I've known.
I'm an old woman now and nature is cruel —
Tis her jest to make old age look like a fool.
The body it crumbles, grace and vigour depart,
There is now a stone where I once had a heart,
But inside this old carcase a young girl still dwells,
And now and again my battered heart swells.
I remember the joys, I remember the pain
And I'm loving and living life over again.
I think of the years all too few, gone too fast,

And accept the stark fact that nothing can last.
So open your eyes, nurse, open and see
Not a crabbit old woman, look closer, see ME!

For further reading:

BLYTHE, R. 1981. *The View in Winter*. London: Penguin.
BUTLER, R. N. & LEWIS M. I. 1983. *Ageing and Mental Health*. St. Louis: Mosby.
KASTENBAUM, R. 1979. *Growing Old*. London: Harper & Row.

2

Physical Ageing and the Presentation of Illness

The changes in the body with advancing years reveal a common pattern. There is some loss of water and a reduction in lean body mass (total weight of fat free tissue). Most of the organs become smaller and show some decline in function. For example, from about the age of 60 the brain begins to shrink and is 5 to 10 per cent smaller by the ninth decade. Its blood flow decreases in proportion. The heart muscle loses some of its power and the cardiac output falls by about a quarter. The chest wall becomes more rigid and the lungs lose some of their elasticity. The pressure of oxygen in the arterial blood falls by about 20 per cent.

The blood flow through the liver and kidneys decreases by about half between the ages of 30 and 75. This is the reason why the older patient takes longer to metabolise and excrete drugs and usually requires his medicine in smaller doses. The immune system undergoes important changes also. These are thought to be the reason for the older patient's predisposition to certain infections and perhaps to the fact that the risk of cancer increases steadily with age.

One feature of ageing is its great variability. The changes vary in degree from person to person and from organ to organ within the same individual. But the trend is always in the same direction. The function of the body is sufficient for life but the reserves are reduced. The older patient is compelled to go more slowly and his powers of adaptation become confined within progressively narrower limits. The older a person is the greater the chance that he will die. In extreme old age death may be brought about by relatively minor illness or injury which would not have been fatal in a younger person.

Cellular ageing

The reduced function of the organs of the body results from a loss of the cells from which they are composed. Not all cells behave in the same way.

Some cells like those of the brain and central nervous system are present at birth and do not divide or reproduce. As an individual matures, however, dendrites, the branching processes which connect one nerve cell with another, become more numerous and complex. In old age this process goes into reverse, and the branching decreases (Fig. 1). In certain areas of the brain up to 50 per cent of nerve cells disappear.

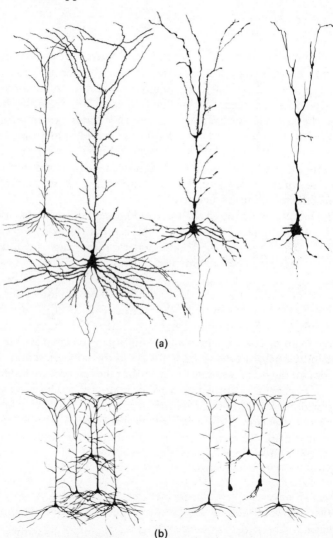

(a)

(b)

Fig. 1 (a) Change in neurones with advancing age. Courtesy of Professor A. B. Scheibel and Churchill Livingstone.

(b) Young and old neuronal networks. Courtesy of Professor A. B. Scheibel and Raven Press.

Other cells, like those of the liver and kidney, rarely divide but can do so if the need arises, for example after surgical removal. Others again have a short life and are constantly replaced. Red blood cells have a life of 120 days, white blood cells of about one week. The cells of the intestinal mucosa are renewed every two or three days.

How cellular ageing takes place is not known. It may be related to DNA, the chemical in the cell nucleus which determines its function and ensures, when the cell divides, that the new cell is a perfect copy of the old. It may be that in the nervous system, for example, the DNA carries a programme for cell life of a predetermined length and the cell dies when this is completed. Or it may be that when cells divide frequently, mutation occurs and the copies become imperfect until they are no longer viable. Or it may be that the lymphocytes, the cells that normally make antibodies to protect against foreign substances, produce auto-antibodies against the cells of the person's own body. Much more research is needed to discover which, if any, of these theories is correct.

Clinical evidence of ageing

From the clinical point of view the main features of ageing are an altered physical appearance, a gradual loss of mobility, and impairment of the special senses.

Physical appearance

One of the most obvious features of the older patient is greying of the hair, which also tends to become sparse and coarser in texture. Baldness of course is common in men, but even in women there may be a considerable thinning of the hair.

The skin acquires a dry, wrinkled appearance. Warts of various kinds are common, particularly on the trunk. There is usually some loss of subcutaneous fat. This deprives the older patient of a useful cushion to cover the bony prominences, and it may be one of the reasons why old people are intolerant of colds and draughts. Sometimes it raises problems deciding where to give an injection.

The blood vessels of the skin are more fragile in old age. The loss of subcutaneous tissue in the hands makes the veins unduly prominent. Spontaneous rupture of blood vessels leads to patches of senile purpura on the back of the hands and forearms. These are not harmful in any way though they may alarm the patient. His family may mistakenly take them as evidence that he has been roughly handled.

The face

The face, and indeed the body generally, has a shrunken look. The eyes may lack lustre due to the arcus senilis, an opaque ring which forms outside the iris, but has no effect on the function of the eye. The pupils are smaller. The wizened look of the face is partly due to loss of subcutaneous fat, but mainly it is due to atrophy of the bones of the face. The altered shape of the jaws in old age makes it harder to wear dentures comfortably. Where the old person has teeth of his own, these always appear to be unduly prominent because of the recession of the gums from the neck of the tooth. Hence the expression 'long in the tooth', a traditional phrase to describe a person as old. With all these changes in the mouth, speech is often slower and less distinct.

The body

The body generally tends to be somewhat bent and all old people lose a little height. This is partly due to muscular weakness, but the main cause is osteoporosis, or atrophy of the bones. As old age advances there is loss of bone substance and the skeleton tends to give way under strain. The thoracic spine in particular becomes increasingly bowed The bones in old age are more fragile and break more readily, often after quite slight degrees of force. Fractures, especially of the neck of the femur, are a common problem in the elderly.

At the same time as calcium is lost from the bones of an old person, it tends to be laid down in new places; calcification occurs in the costal cartilages, the wall of the aorta, the thyroid, the trachea and the bronchi. The reason for this is unknown.

Mobility

The older patient has less energy and is not as agile as he was in his youth. A general slowing-up of movement is the rule. Painful feet may be an additional handicap. The gait becomes stiff and the steps tend to be short. Dressing and getting in and out of bed may become difficult. This reduced mobility may be due to changes in the nervous system, in the joints and in the muscles. In the nervous system the loss of cells from the brain and spinal cord leads to a slowing and failure of co-ordination in bodily movements. Balance becomes less good and there is a greater tendency to fall. There may be some loss of skill in the upper limbs and a tremor of the hands is not uncommon.

Some degenerative changes in the joints are universal in the older patient. They affect particularly the cartilage of the knees and hips. The joints may become stiff and can sometimes be felt to creak like a rusty hinge. Muscle power and bulk decreases even in the healthiest old people. The 'shrunk shank' of the old person has been noted since the days of Shakespeare. These changes may not be as inevitable as they have seemed hitherto. Research in the USSR has shown that much immobility may be due to stagnation and can be prevented by exercise. The body needs to be used if it is to be kept in trim. Movement is life, and activity can be maintained by a regular programme of walking and exercise. The 'daily dozen' may be the best prescription against the ravages of old age.

The special senses

The special senses of sight, hearing and smell are all liable to deteriorate in old age and may play an important part in increasing the difficulties of the older patient.

Eyesight is at its most perfect as early as the age of ten. Thereafter the lens, which enables the eye to focus clearly on near or distant objects, slowly loses its elasticity. This is not at first detectable except with special instruments and usually does not cause any inconvenience until middle age or later when the patient finds he can no longer see for close work without the aid of spectacles, a condition known as presbyopia.

An old person's glasses are vital to him and must never be taken away. Sight should be tested every two years.

Hearing too is at its peak in childhood and slowly declines with age, especially in the capacity to detect high frequency sounds. By the age of 60 most people have lost three-quarters of their capacity to hear high frequency sounds. This is fortunately not very disabling, because ordinary speech consists of sounds of a quite low frequency which can still be appreciated in old age. Even so, deafness is a common problem for the older patient.

The sense of smell, never very acute in humans as compared with animals, also deteriorates with age, and with it the sense of taste. This does not mean that the older patient is incapable of enjoying his food, but he may like to be free with the condiments and the sauce bottle. An impaired sense of smell may make him less quick to smell burning for example and his life is thus made a little more hazardous.

The older patient in illness

Although there are no diseases peculiar to old age, illness in the older patient commonly reveals a number of special features.

Multiple pathology

In old age it is the rule rather than the exception for the patient to suffer from several diseases at once. In acute illness it is usually clear which disease is dominant, but some account must be taken of the others. A patient with a stroke, for example, may well be handicapped also by cataracts which limit his vision, heart disease which limits his capacity for effort, a urinary infection which increases the risk of incontinence and osteoarthrosis of the hips or knees which further restricts his mobility. All these, as well as the stroke, demand treatment and affect his rehabilitation.

Confusion

In the older patient the stability of the brain is precariously balanced, probably because of the usual loss of nerve cells. The function of the brain is readily upset by any kind of bodily disturbance, and a sudden onset of confusion is one of the commonest indications of physical illness in old age. It is comparable to the delirium which may accompany grave illness in the younger patient but occurs much more frequently and for lesser causes. In a patient without previous mental impairment the onset of confusion suggests serious physical illness, but in those whose minds are already beginning to fail, confusion may be provoked by quite minor bodily disturbances. Such reactions are often short-lived and subside as soon as the physical disorder is corrected. They are very common and may be seen in as many as one patient in three in a geriatric ward.

Immobility and falls

Falls and immobility when the patient goes off his legs are among the commonest reasons for the older patient's admission to hospital.

And often he is confused into the bargain. Like confusion, immobility and falls are a non-specific manifestation of disease. The underlying cause may be an infection, a myocardial infarct, a stroke, or any one of a hundred other causes. It may also be the effect of drugs.

Loss of pain sensation

The older patient often has a diminished sense of pain. This makes life less uncomfortable for him but it increases the risk that he may injure himself. For example he may burn his shins by sitting too close to the fire. He may injure his leg against a bed cradle. He may bruise his arms against a safety side or locker. Hot water bottles are a special danger.

Even serious injuries like fractures may not be obvious. An old person who breaks the neck of his femur, for example, may have only mild discomfort even though he cannot walk. In abdominal emergencies such as acute appendicitis there may be little pain or tenderness until the disease is far advanced. Myocardial infarction in younger patients is invariably associated with crushing chest pain. In the great majority of elderly patients it is painless.

Temperature regulation

The regulation of body temperature is less efficient in the older patient, and fever is less obvious and less severe. But an illness which will provoke a sharp rise in temperature in a younger patient may in the elderly cause only a small rise or none at all. Rigors are exceptional and usually indicate a urinary or gallbladder infection. If an old person seems unwell there can be no reassurance in the fact that his temperature is normal. The pulse and respiration will often be a better guide to his condition. The defective temperature regulation of the older patient is also seen in his reaction to cold when his body temperature may fall below normal in the condition known as hypothermia.

Dehydration

Old people probably have an impaired sense of thirst. They readily become too weak or apathetic to drink. Those who are mentally disturbed may refuse food and drink but naturally continue to lose fluid in the urine and sweat and are thus very likely to become dehydrated. It is remarkable how a sick old person may begin to improve after some intravenous or subcutaneous fluid.

Reaction to drugs

The older patient is very sensitive to drugs and harmful side effects are common. Drugs are more slowly metabolised in the liver and are excreted more slowly by the kidneys. Thus many medicines must be given in smaller doses than would have been appropriate in earlier life. Moreover one drug may react with another in unexpected ways and the multiple diseases often present tempt the doctor into prescribing too many drugs. The precarious stability of the brain makes confusion a common side effect of numerous drugs, especially hypnotics, tranquillisers and antidepressants.

Need to preserve mobility

Many of the illnesses which affect the older patient cause prolonged disability. There is, therefore, a tendency to think that the older patient has delayed powers of recovery. This is not so. Wounds heal and fractures mend almost as quickly in the old as in the young, and many old people can throw off an acute infection or an attack of heart failure quite readily. On the other hand old people deteriorate quickly if they are kept inactive and especially if they are kept in bed.

The patient must always be viewed as a whole and his future as a functioning human being must never be forgotten. It is vital to preserve his mobility. It is, for example, no service to a patient with heart disease to keep him in bed so long that when he gets up he has lost the ability to walk. Future disabilities must, as far as possible, be foreseen and prevented. This is largely done by nursing the patient out of bed, by helping him to his feet as soon as possible and by encouraging all forms of activity of mind and body. The deliberate assistance of the patient's own healing power underlies the whole process of geriatric rehabilitation.

For further reading:

COMFORT, A. 1977. *A Good Age*. London: Mitchell Beazley.

CONI, N., DAVISON, W. & WEBSTER, S. 1985. *Ageing: The Facts*. Oxford: Blackwell.

HODKINSON, H. M. 1976. *Common Symptoms of Disease in the Elderly*. Oxford: Blackwell.

3
Retirement, Money and Housing

Each year about half a million people retire from work, a step
which marks the beginning of a new way of life that may last twenty
or thirty years. For many people the age of retirement is fixed by the
conditions of their employment, often 60 for women and 65 for
men. Some people are able to retire earlier on a reduced pension
or to work on for an increased one, but only the self-employed
have complete freedom to go on working or to retire as they
wish.

Retirement problems

The central problem of the 9.5 million retired people in Great
Britain is the maintenance of activity and interest on a reduced
income. Fortunately most of them can expect good health and find
retirement happy and rewarding.

But not all. Many men and some women feel work to be their
primary interest. From their job they obtain the money, status and
associations which make life worth living. To them retirement
involves an unwelcome change. Some fail to adjust and are unable
to find satisfaction in their new role. Such people may become ill
physically or mentally, a few even to the point of suicide. The
housewife however, far from retiring, has new adjustments to
make with her husband at home all day, a situation which may
enhance a happy marriage or place intolerable strains upon a shaky
one.

However, retirement is often a time of opportunity, development and new friendships. There are a multiplicity of clubs, societies
and facilities for adult education. It is even possible to take a degree
through the Open University. And for those who prefer work
rather than study there may be part-time employment and
innumerable opportunities to help others as a good neighbour or as a
member of a voluntary society. The recently retired are now the
country's major source of voluntary workers and the opportunities
to find self-fulfilment are legion. No wonder the French refer to life
after retirement as 'the third age'.

Preparation for retirement

To retire successfully requires preparation. Pre-retirement education, at present only offered to 6 per cent of retirees, has proved
its value. Topics covered in pre-retirement courses include finance,
education, health, hobbies and do-it-yourself. There is a monthly
magazine, *Choice*, specifically for the retired.

   Pre-retirement education has been pioneered for about twenty
years by the Pre-retirement Association (19 Undine Street, London
SW17 8PP). This organisation works closely with the Trade Union
Congress and the Industrial Society. Retirement courses are
provided now by many individual organisations and firms as well as
by local education authorities. In some areas there are 'Retirement
Councils' which promote courses, craft centres and employment
bureaux.

Finance

The financial circumstances of retired people vary as much as
those in employment. Two-thirds report that they have enough to
manage. Even in retirement a few, about one in ten married couples
and single men but only one in thirty single women, are well off.
This is usually because of a generous occupational pension or private
income from investments.

   On average however, retired people have half the income of
those at work. They are less likely to own a car, a telephone, a
washing machine or central heating, but nearly everyone has a
television set and three out of four a refrigerator.

   The greatest financial difficulties are faced by women on their
own, widowed, single or divorced. Their problem is widespread
since 80 per cent of women over 75 have no husband.

   For both men and women income decreases with age. The
income of those over 75 is almost 30 per cent less than that of the
recently retired. One in five men and one in three women over 75
need supplementary benefit, as do half of those over 85. Such people
are no longer able to supplement their income with odd jobs and are
likely to have exhausted their savings. Bed linen, clothes and
furniture wear out and have to be replaced. There may be a need to
pay for help in the house and garden. The smaller a person's income
the greater the proportion of it that must be spent on the basic
necessities of life. An unexpected bill may cause anxiety with less to
spend on food and fuel.

State retirement pension

The state retirement pension is one of the benefits for which people pay by compulsory deductions from their earnings throughout working life. The employer too is required by law to make a contribution to the National Insurance Fund for each person he employs. At present women qualify for the retirement pension at 60 and men at 65, an arrangement which lacks both logic and justice since women live longer than men. In most other European countries and in the United States both sexes retire at the same age, ranging from 67 in Denmark to 60 in France. Britain is likely to follow suit eventually and the Government has declared its intention to work towards a common retirement age with some choice for individuals. Rising unemployment may result in a lowering of pensionable age for men.

Since it was introduced by Lloyd George in 1908 the state retirement pension has been paid at a flat rate. In 1985 this was £38.30 for a single person and £61.30 for a married couple. Pensions are linked to average earnings, but not prices, so they are not fully protected against inflation. The pension goes up by 7.5 per cent each year if a person postpones his retirement. A five year deferment increases the value of the pension by 37.5 per cent.

State Earning Related Pension Scheme (SERPS)

A new development in 1978 was the introduction of an earnings related pension to supplement the flat rate state pension. This, it is intended, will largely replace supplementary benefit. At present the weekly maximum is £3.45 but by the end of the century when the scheme is fully mature a married man with national average earnings will retire with a pension for himself and his wife of half his earnings at retirement. However, in 1985 the government proposed to abolish SERPS after the year 2001, and to replace it by private arrangements.

Occupational pensions

Nearly 4 million people now receive an occupational pension from their previous employers. Eventually it is estimated some 10 million people will benefit in this way. About 40 per cent of retired people enjoy some form of occupational pension, but in only 6 per cent is it the principal source of income. Occupational pensions are more likely to be enjoyed by those under 75 and by men rather than by women.

Supplementary Benefit (Income Support)

Earnings related schemes are largely for the future and the present retirement pension is not enough to live on by itself. If a person's other resources are inadequate he is entitled to claim a supplementary pension from the Department of Health and Social Security (DHSS) to bring his income to a guaranteed level. His right to this is unaffected by having up to £3000 in savings and by owning the house in which he lives. The amounts payable are laid down in regulations approved by Parliament.

1.7 million people claimed supplementary benefit in 1978 but it was estimated by the DHSS that a further 600 000 would have been entitled had they applied. The reasons why people fail to apply for a pension to which they are entitled is probably due to a feeling which still lingers, however erroneously, that supplementary benefit is a charity and not a right. Moreover it depends on a means test and many people are naturally reluctant to disclose their financial circumstances. For all these reasons the government proposed in 1985 to rename Supplementary Benefit 'Income Support'.

Attendance Allowance

The national retirement pension is related to age and previous employment. Supplementary pension is means tested and designed to prevent extreme poverty. But there is also an allowance based on disability and the need for care. This is the Attendance Allowance, introduced in 1971. It is a tax-free benefit payable regardless of income to people who need constant attention for mental or physical disability. There are two weekly rates, £30.60 for those needing care throughout the twenty-four hours and £20.45 for those needing care by day or night only. Three hundred thousand people, most of them elderly, received the Attendance Allowance in 1981.

The allowance is payable to those living at home or in private old people's homes and nursing homes. Those in hospital or local authority homes are not eligible. The allowance enables some people to choose care in the private sector, a fact of growing importance as the statutory services are coming under increasing pressure from the rise in numbers of old people and by cuts in public spending.

Invalid Care Allowance

Since 1976 the Attendance Allowance has been complemented by the Invalid Care Allowance. This goes to men and single women who are unable to work because they are at home looking after someone in receipt of the Attendance Allowance. In 1982 this allowance was worth £23.00. Married women are excluded from this allowance which many feel to be unjust. This is likely to change following an EEC decision in 1985. Only 7000 people received the Invalid Care Allowance in 1981.

Housing Finance

An old person on a low income living in rented accommodation may be entitled to a rent allowance from the local authority even though he does not qualify for a supplementary pension.

Rate rebates are available both to tenants and owner-occupiers. In 1978 800 000 pensioners claimed rent allowances and 1.8 million rate rebates.

Grants are also available from the local authorities for home improvements such as bathrooms, hot water systems and insulation. All these arrangements are currently under review.

Private income

All financial arrangements mentioned above are ways in which the state or the local authority helps a retired person to maintain his income. But one retired person in three also has a private income from savings, investment or insurance. In 4 per cent this is the principal source of their income. More men than women have private income.

Concessionary prices

Retired people, because of their large numbers, are an important market for manufacturers and the providers of services, who may woo them with various cut price offers. The Senior Citizen's Railcard is well known, as are concessionary bus and coach fares. Sometimes admission charges to theatres, cinemas and exhibitions are reduced to pensioners. Hairdressers offer reduced charges to pensioners on certain days. All this helps to offset the expense of buying in small quantities which is often a problem for elderly people.

Pensions in the future

Pensions, it has been said, represent a contract between the generations. Today's pensioners are largely funded by the taxes paid by today's workers.

By the end of this century the total number of pensioners will not increase though there will be many more very old people among them. The numbers in the work force will increase. Today there are 2.77 workers for every pensioner. In 2001 there will be 2.99, so things should be better. By 2030, however, if people continue to have very small families there will be only 2.04 workers for every pensioner and things may be very difficult indeed.

Housing

When he first retires a person's housing may be no more than a matter of convenience and many people move to the coast or to the country. Later however, if the person becomes infirm or loses his partner, the availability of family and friends becomes of crucial importance. Given suitable housing and appropriate help, most old people can live an independent life even if very disabled and nine out of ten do so. But without suitable housing their problems may become overwhelming.

Flats, preferably with a lift, or bungalows suit many old people best. Ideally they should be on a bus route and close to churches and shops rather than in a quiet backwater. Most old people prefer to watch the passing scene and transport facilities are important to them. They need to see and meet the young so their homes should not be all grouped together but distributed among other dwellings. Ground floor flats, although they have many advantages, have disadvantages too, including noise, some loss of privacy, and a greater risk of burglary or vandalism. Sometimes the rent and insurance premiums are higher also.

Supported independence

Some people who have younger relatives may prefer a supported type of independence. For them and their relatives buildings have been designed with separate but adjoining accommodation. These are often known as 'Granny Annexes'. They enable the old person to maintain independence and privacy while help and companionship are at hand if needed.

Sheltered housing

Another kind of supported independence is provided by sheltered housing. This usually consists of bungalows or flatlets with a resident

Warden. Her duty is to keep a friendly eye on the residents and to summon help when needed — a bell or call system connects each flat with the warden. There is often a common room where the residents may meet if they wish.

Wardens were originally supposed to keep an eye on the residents in return for free accommodation and a low salary. It was not anticipated that there would be so many calls upon them. However as time has advanced residents in sheltered housing have become frailer and warden cover has had to be extended. It is now not uncommon for two or three wardens to be appointed providing care around the clock. An alternative and more economical idea is to provide peripatetic wardens, particularly at night. Sheltered housing units are connected to a central call point by radio or telephone and a warden who will visit by car is available to be summoned at any time, including the night.

Local authority housing

In Great Britain local authorities have a duty to provide housing for those in need, and one-third of the elderly are housed by them. The local authorities are the major providers of sheltered housing for frail and disabled people. The purpose built old people's flats and bungalows are an increasing feature of the local authority's scheme and some of them have a warden. Local authority housing standards have risen in the last few years and much of their accommodation is of excellent quality. Unfortunately there is always a waiting list and it will take many years to satisfy the ever expanding need.

Housing Associations

Almhouses, started by individual charitable donors, were the earliest form of special housing for the elderly and some are still in existence. It is possible also for people to form a housing association through which they can borrow money to provide accommodation for themselves or their tenants. Schemes may include warden supervision. One of the greatest difficulties faced by any housing association is to keep down the cost so that the rents are within the means of those most in need.

Private tenancies

About one old person in six lives as the tenant of a private landlord. The standards of privately rented accommodation vary

from luxury flats to squalid bed-sitting rooms in decaying tene-
ments. Because of their poor economic circumstances, often
aggravated by a loss of business acumen, many old people live in
unsatisfactory housing. A third of a million have no bath, kitchen or
indoor lavatory. But some people prefer to live at a low rent in
housing that they have been used to all their lives rather than face the
disruption that improvements would involve.

Private ownership

Almost half of all old people own their own homes. An old
person may cling to his house when it has become too large for him
or has never been modernised. It may be possible to remain in
familiar surroundings, however, if he converts his house into flats
with the help of an Improvement Grant from the local authority or
by a loan from a bank, building society or insurance company.

Safety in the home

Suitable housing for the elderly is important also from the point
of view of safety. Each year there are some 9,000 fatal home
accidents and more deaths occur in the home than on the roads. The
great majority result from falls, but there are also deaths from burns.
Some of these disasters could be avoided by better planning. The
most dangerous places are the stairs, the kitchen and the bathroom.
Many falls occur around the bed.

Stairs

If possible an old person should live in a flat or bungalow where
there are no stairs. If this cannot be, the staircase should be well lit
and equipped with a double handrail. A loose mat should never be
placed at the foot or the head of the stairs and nothing should ever be
left on them. The stair carpet should be firmly fixed. Any odd steps
or door sills should be picked out in white paint.

Kitchen

Kitchen cupboards should not be too high. No one should
have to stand on a chair to reach them. Cooking should be done on
electricity or gas. Solid fuel involves more work than most old

people can undertake, while paraffin is dangerous because of the risk of fire. The cooking and work surfaces should be at the same height with the oven alongside and not underneath the hot plate. Many people find it difficult to stoop down to a low oven. If they lose their balance while holding a hot dish with both hands, they cannot save themselves and risk burns as well as a fall. Gas cookers should have self-lighting taps.

Bathroom

To get in and out of a bath is difficult and dangerous for many old people. It is safer to use a shower, but this is not popular in Great Britain. A tub bath needs handrails of which there are many varieties (see p. 166). The lavatory also needs appropriately placed handrails and for some people a raised lavatory seat is an advantage (see p. 219).

Other safety points

Central heating is ideal. If fires are used they should be enclosed by firmly fixed guards. A clock or mirror should never be placed on a mantelpiece above an open fire. Electric blankets should be serviced regularly and over-blankets are preferable if there is any danger of incontinence. Bedside lamps and other electrical appliances should be placed so that there are no long flexes to trip over. Electric power points should be at table height not floor level. Frayed carpets should be repaired or replaced. Lever door handles are easier to turn than door knobs. Window controls should be accessible and easy to manipulate. All medicines should be clearly labelled in large writing and kept in a safe place. Gas and electricity coin meters should be accessible and in a good light.

Minor repairs

Minor repairs can often be done for old people by volunteers from a youth organisation, Age Concern or a church group.

Emergency call systems

An important aspect of home safety is the ability of the resident to seek help in an emergency. A call system to the warden is a key feature of sheltered housing. Many systems, none of them perfect, are available. The simplest and cheapest of these is a walking stick to thump the wall or floor and alert the family or neighbour. Some people carry a whistle.

Alarm bells and flashing lights outside the front door have proved unacceptable. They advertise the old person's vulnerability. Is the front door to be kept unlocked? Or what is to be done with the key?

A better system was introduced by the Borough of Stockport in 1978. This used a short wave radio transmitter to link the old person with a central control station. The system is flexible and is easy to operate. It can be installed or removed quickly. This makes it useful as a temporary expedient in the weeks following return home from hospital. The system does not allow two-way speech. All alarm calls, including many false ones, have to be followed up by a mobile warden.

Two-way speech is possible through a telephone, preferably with a bedside extension. Departments of Social Services can install telephones in houses of handicapped people but they have used their powers sparingly because of the expense. Moreover the telephone has its limitations. If the owner has a stroke or falls down he may not be able to reach the instrument.

The most sophisticated alarms are body-worn aids containing a radio transmitter which activates, directly or via a telephone linc, an alarm at a central point. The operator or a computer then telephones a number of previously identified contact persons, one of whom will visit to see what has happened. These alarms are not expensive to install but there is also a monitoring charge and, of course, the expense of the telephone as well. One new system incorporates an intercom so that the patient can be told directly that this call has been received.

Good neighbours

All these systems depend ultimately on someone being alert to receive the signal and respond to it. The best support of all for the frail old person living alone is his good neighbour. Someone who will notice whether the milk has been brought in and the curtains drawn each day, and who will make enquiries if they are not, is worth all the microchips and electronics in the world.

Gaining co-operation

The points suggested will not be acceptable to the old person unless he himself becomes convinced of their importance. If this vital factor is ignored the safety devices will not be used and the new cooker will stand idly in the kitchen while the old lady continues to cook on a paraffin stove as she did before.

Access for the disabled

Public buildings as well as homes need to be made safe and accessible for the elderly. Two-thirds of all disabled people are over 65 and the proportion rises with advancing age. Thus facilities designed to help disabled people are of particular importance to the elderly. These include ramps, handrails and lifts in public buildings, toilets for those in wheelchairs and those with walking aids. The orange badge which allows parking in restricted areas is available from social service departments to motorists on production of a medical certificate. Buses and coaches are being developed to allow easier access for the disabled. The London Underground is impossible, but more modern systems elsewhere are designed with the needs of the handicapped, including wheelchair users, in mind.

For further reading:

BUTLER, A. & TINKER, A. 1983. *Housing Alternatives for the Elderly*. University of Leeds.

BUTLER, A. & OLDMAN, C. 1981. *Alarm Systems for the Elderly. Report of a workshop held at the University of Leeds*. University of Leeds.

CASEY, J. 1983. *Your Housing in Retirement*. London: Age Concern England.

DHSS. 1978. *A Happier Old Age*. HMSO.

DHSS. 1981. *Growing Older*. HMSO.

EBBETT, A. 1984. *Your Rights: for Pensioners*. Age Concern.

EVES, A. V. 1984. *Money and Your Retirement* (book and cassette). Choice Publications.

4
The Older Patient at Home

Most old people live in their own homes. Two out of five live with their spouse, one in eight with their children.

Only 6 per cent of all those over 65 are in any kind of institution. As age advances, however, the likelihood of living in some form of residential care increases.

Two to three per cent of men and women aged 65–74 are in some form of hospital or home as are 10 per cent of men and 15 per cent of women over 80. Thus in even the most vulnerable group, women over 80, at least four out of five live at home and many of these live alone.

Living alone

The number of people living alone in Britain more than doubled between 1961 and 1981. Now more than four million people live alone and many of them are elderly. One-quarter of the old people in Britain has neither spouse nor children and their number is increasing. One-third of those over 65 now lives alone and more than half of those over 75.

Most old people however prefer to live alone and value their independence. Many have frequent contact with their family and friends. If they become infirm they may need help but they are self-sufficient emotionally.

Loneliness

Not everyone who lives alone is lonely. It is quite possible for an old person to feel lonely or homesick even in a residential home. Loneliness is however a special burden to those who are isolated. These are often people with personality difficulties which prevent them from forming satisfactory social relationships. Throughout life they have antagonised their relatives and neighbours. They may be aggressively independent, repelling all offers of help. Occasionally compulsory admission to hospital by Court Order (Section 47) may be the only way of getting the help that is so badly needed. Many such isolates are found as long-stay residents in geriatric wards or old people's homes where they may continue to have difficulty in fitting in.

Bereavement

Another group of lonely people are those who have been bereaved. Bereavement, and the grief which it causes, is a common experience in old age, but that does not make it any less painful. The longer an old person lives the more likely he is to experience death among his family, friends and contemporaries. The loss of a spouse is the commonest form of bereavement and almost all women will experience this eventually. The loss of an adult son or daughter, especially one on whom an old person has come to depend for help, may be particularly devastating. The loss of one's home, or the loss of one's physical integrity and mobility through a stroke or surgical amputation, even the loss of a pet, may also provoke a severe grief reaction.

Most old people after bereavement eventually adjust to their changed circumstances, but it may take a year or two.

Phases of grief

The normal pattern of grieving is recognised as having three main phases. The first is one of shock and stunned disbelief. This may be overwhelming if the bereaved person is not prepared for the intensity of the emotions he may experience. He may feel numbed, exhausted, apathetic, or he may be driven to purposeless over-activity. This phase commonly lasts until the funeral which serves to give public recognition to the changed status of the bereaved person.

The second phase is one of prolonged emotional turmoil. The bereaved person may experience a welter of emotions, misery, resentment, fears of the future, guilt, hostility and desolation. Older people are particularly likely to suffer from physical symptoms also at this time.

Eventually after a period of months or years, intense grief dies away leading to the third phase, that of resolution, when the bereaved person comes to terms with his loss and begins to rebuild his life.

These stages are not always clear cut in old people, especially when there is mental impairment. In some people grief appears to be less intense, but those who cannot express it may become ill, mentally or physically, and perhaps follow their partner to an early grave. In others grief may fail to resolve, persisting for a long time in the form of chronic anger, hostility and apathy.

Others again may take on a new lease of life after bereavement, especially if the care of the dying spouse has been a great burden. Old people's response to bereavement is as varied as human personality.

Support for the old person at home

Many people under 75, whether they live alone or with a spouse, manage to remain entirely independent. They make no demands on anybody but they are vulnerable in case of accident or illness. However, by the age of 85 one in five is housebound and most of those who can still get around find themselves in need of help.

Help from relatives

If he has relatives the old person may receive much support from them. It is not unusual for a very frail person to be maintained at home by a married daughter living nearby who visits two or three times a day to do all the cooking, cleaning and shopping, and to give such personal care as may be necessary. Sometimes the work is shared between several members of the family including the grand-children. In other cases a friendly neighbour will provide a great deal of assistance.

Home Help Service

Where there are no relatives available or where they are unable to do all that is needed, the old person may require support from the Home Help Service. In some cases the old person may depend entirely on this kind of help. In others the Home Help Service may be used to supplement care provided by the family and friends. About one person in seven over the age of 75 receives home help.

The home help, sometimes called a home care worker, will undertake any of the tasks normally performed by the housewife. She will prepare meals, shop, collect the pension, clean the house, do the laundry, and empty the commode. She may also offer more personal care, such as helping the old person to wash, to dress and to do her hair.

At present less than 10 per cent of the elderly receive home help though the proportion rises to 16 per cent for those over 75 and 27 per cent for those over 85. The amount of help offered varies from an hour or two once a week to more intensive schemes providing visits seven days a week. The home help may even sleep in at times of crisis.

Home help is not provided free and the amount required and the money the patient must pay are determined by the home help organiser.

All this takes time and in hospital it often happens that a patient requiring home help cannot be discharged immediately. But sometimes the process can be speeded up. The East Sussex County Council, for example, has pioneered the Post Hospital Immediate Care Scheme (PHICS). This provides immediate help at a fixed and very low charge for two weeks and enables an old person to go home from hospital as soon as he is ready.

Meals on Wheels

The provision of cooked meals can be a problem for an old person, especially if he is housebound. He may lack the energy to plan his meals, and perhaps find it too much trouble to cook. A meal may be cooked for him by the home help or by a friendly neighbour, but an important provider is the Meals on Wheels Service. Pioneered by the Women's Royal Voluntary Service (WRVS), the Meals on Wheels Service is financed by the Social Services Department and the meals are still often delivered by volunteers. About one in twenty of those over 75 receive meals on wheels.

Meals on wheels are seldom available at weekends or on Bank Holidays. It is usually only possible for a person to be visited three or four times a week. This is not enough for those in greatest need. There is seldom any choice of menu or provision for special diets. But in spite of its limitations the service is much appreciated.

Friendly visiting

Many old people are lonely. They can often be helped by regular friendly visiting, a service which is provided by voluntary organisations such as Age Concern, WRVS and the churches. The most valuable part of visiting is to show interest and friendship. Some visitors may perform small services such as writing letters, changing library books or taking the old person out. The successful visitor will encourage the old person to talk and will manage to convey his genuine interest and concern while avoiding any hint of patronage or condescension. Such simple acts of friendship give an old person a sense of his continued significance as a human being. They raise his morale and are an important antidote to loneliness.

Holidays

Older people, like younger ones, need holidays. Those in good health can usually make their own arrangements, either alone or in a party, and many seaside towns offer out-of-season reduced rates for pensioners. Old people's clubs often arrange group holidays for their members and Age Concern publishes a useful booklet, *Holidays for the Elderly*. SAGA Holidays of Folkestone specialise in travel arrangements for older people. Social Services Departments can also arrange holidays under the provision of the Chronically Sick and Disabled Persons Act 1970. Some authorities, usually in urban areas, maintain their own holiday homes at the seaside.

Respite care

Disabled old people make great demands on those who care for them and the carers themselves need relief from time to time, to have a holiday or simply to have some hours to themselves. This may be achieved by day care (see p. 75), respite admission to hospital or old people's home (see p. 52) or by a relief service to the home.

Relief care at home can occasionally be provided by special residential home help. Voluntary help in the home to give relief to carers has been pioneered by the Crossroads Scheme and by the Cheshire Foundation. The new Association of Carers is trying to create mutual support and self-help in this field and to put pressure on the local authorities to make shared care between families and social services a reality. The Marie Curie Foundation enables trained nurses to spend the night at the homes of patients with cancer.

Laundry service

Where an incontinent old person is being nursed at home there may be a severe laundry problem. To meet this some districts have established a special laundry service for the incontinent, but this is tending to be replaced by the increased use of disposable incontinence pads. These however create their own problems of disposal and incineration.

Health care at home

The Primary Health Care Team, a most valuable development made possible by the National Health Service, plays an important part in enabling the older patient to remain at home. The team is now likely to work from a health centre or purpose-built surgery. Regular meetings, formal and informal, help to keep the team together in pursuit of common objectives.

The general practitioner

More old people are in touch with the general practitioner and his team than with any other source of help. The general practitioner or deputy is always available and will visit those who are too ill or too handicapped to get to the surgery. Ninety-five per cent of old people live at home and depend on their family doctor for medical care and support. He looks after his patients when they go into an old people's home or nursing home and sometimes cares for them in hospital also if there are general practitioner beds. The round-the-clock accessibility of the general practitioner and the continuity of care he provides are among the most appreciated features of the National Health Service.

Community nurses

Nurse members of the Primary Health Care Team have much to contribute. At least half their time is spent with the elderly and much more in retirement areas. All now receive special training.

The registered community nurse

Registered General Nurses (RGN) working in the community have successfully completed six months of college based training followed by a period of supervised practice and have been awarded the District Nurses Certificate (DNCert).

The community sister or charge nurse, like her hospital counterpart, leads a team of nurses. Her job is to assess the nursing needs of her patients and to plan their care, using all the resources of the nursing team and delegating where appropriate. The training of learners and other nurses in the team is an important part of her duties.

The enrolled community nurse

The state enrolled community nurse has her own group of patients under the general direction of the community sister. It is recommended that she should receive four months' training, though this is not yet compulsory.

The nursing auxiliary

The nursing auxiliary is an important member of the team, working closely with the trained nurses. She is likely to receive in-service training.

Pattern of work

Community nurses give care in acute, terminal or long-term illness. They have a special part to play in the rehabilitation of the older patient in co-operation with the domiciliary physiotherapist or occupational therapist. Where relatives or friends are available the nurse will show them how to lift and teach them other aspects of care. She has access to nursing aids such as back rests, commodes, incontinence appliances and other disposables. She will be concerned also with those recently discharged from hospital and good communication between the hospital and the community nursing team is vital (see p. 75).

New developments in community nursing have improved the care of the older patient. The twilight service enables an evening visit to be made, allowing a more normal bedtime for those who need help to get to bed. The night service provides visits through the night to give care and treatment especially to the terminally ill.

Health visitors

Like community nurses, health visitors are part of a Primary Health Care Team and work closely with the general practitioner. They are registered nurses and midwives with an additional qualification in the preventative and social aspects of health.

The health visitor is concerned with the family at all ages. Her responsibilities include visiting to assess the needs of the older patient and of those who care for him. She may advise on home safety, nutrition and finance. She has an important role as a case finder. If the practice has an age/sex register she will be able to identify and visit those at risk. These include old people who live alone, the recently bereaved, the housebound, the mentally ill and those recently discharged from hospital. Elderly people often attribute their ailments to old age. The health visitor may be able to persuade them that old age and illness are not the same thing and that their disabilities may be improved if they will seek investigation and treatment.

Some health visitors have special responsibility as liaison officers between the hospital and the community. Their duties may include follow-up visits to those who have been discharged and assessment visits to those who have been referred for admission or day hospital treatment.

Specialist nurse advisers

Where there is a comprehensive service for the elderly with mental illness, community psychiatric nurses (CPN) are employed to advise and give support to the older patient and his family. Other specialist nurses have responsibilities in the field of stoma care, pain control or incontinence. These and other specialists provide an expertise invaluable to their colleagues as well as to their patients.

Chiropody

The commonest single disability of the older patient is difficulty in cutting his toenails. Many old people are unable to care for their feet because of stiff hips, poor eyesight or shaky hands. Toenails may become thickened, a condition called onychauxis, or overgrown in fantastic shapes like a ramshorn, known as onychogryposis. Changes in the toenails may prevent the patient from wearing his shoes. Corns, callouses and bunions, which sometimes become infected, may cause pain and immobility. Systemic disorders such as diabetes, arterial disease and rheumatoid arthritis, expose the feet to special hazards. Most chiropodists are in private practice but schemes exist to provide foot care for those who cannot pay. Some chiropodists do essential work at health centres, day centres and hospitals. An increasing number of fully trained chiropodists now work full-time for the National Health Service. There are still too few to meet all needs but the situation is slowly improving.

For further reading:

HEDLEY, R. & NORMAN, A. J. 1982. *Home Help: Key Issues in Service Provision*. Centre for Policy on Ageing.
HUNT, A. 1978. *The Elderly at Home*. HMSO.
NORMAN, A. J. 1980. *Rights and Risk*. Centre for Policy on Ageing.

5
Families and Carers

Many of the problems of the older patient revolve around his family relationships. To understand him properly it is essential to see him not as an isolated individual but as a member of a family.

The changing family

Families are smaller than they used to be. Nowadays the average family has two children but at the beginning of the century most families had five or six. Three generations commonly lived together and it was usual for an unmarried daughter to remain at home and look after her parents. Moreover even in quite modest families there was often domestic help. In these larger households it was possible to provide the care needed for an old person and the hospitals could offer nothing that was not equally well done at home.

Today family patterns of living have changed. Earlier marriage, the more extensive employment of women, the greater mobility of the working population, all make it harder for a family to care for its aged members. Even so more women today are caring for elderly relatives than for children.

Divorce too creates problems for old people. It is still unusual for a marriage to break up in old age but elderly people may be distressed and confused by divorce among their children, probably themselves middle-aged. Remarriage will produce a crop of new in-laws and step-grandchildren with whom the old person may find it hard to build a relationship. Divorce may also create problems of legal access by old people to their grandchildren.

Increased opportunities for education and training may mean that the 'children's' way of life, their interests, their friends, their habits and even their speech are very different from those of their parents. These things can provoke great tension within a family.

Moreover many more people now survive into old age. The average elderly couple can expect that during the last years of their marriage one of them may be physically or mentally frail and housebound.

Family responsibilities

In Great Britain today there is no legal compulsion for the younger generation to support their parents, but a moral obligation to do so is widely accepted. It is often said that the Welfare State has undermined family responsibility and that people no longer look after their aged relatives as they did in the past. There is in fact little evidence of this and those with most experience are constantly impressed with the amount of care which elderly people receive from their families. Difficulties arise when the old person has no relatives, is estranged from them, or when the family has other responsibilities. One old person in three has no relatives within reach. More than one in three has no living children. When they do have younger relatives living nearby, however, old people continue to rely on them. In a recent survey it was found that four out of five old people with living children had at least one member of the family less than half-an-hour away, and saw them frequently. Two-thirds had been helped by their families when they were ill and over half were receiving assistance with their housework. Similar figures were found in Denmark and America. They confirm that the pattern of supported independence is one of the most satisfactory ways of living in old age.

Another study has shown that three-quarters of the most handicapped people in the community are being looked after by their families and that only one-quarter are in any kind of hospital or home. The nurse can confirm this when she sees how disabled are many of the patients coming to hospital to allow their relatives a holiday. Overall only five out of every hundred people over 65 live in any kind of institution. The rest live at home, alone or with their relatives.

Relationships within the family

In any family the children are at first entirely dependent upon their parents, but gradually grow away from them. Later the children leave home to work or marry and set up homes of their own. At this stage the parents may still be middle-aged and the two generations can live independently of one another in a relationship of equality. Finally the older generation may in its turn become dependent upon the young. By this time it is probable that the 'children' will themselves be retired and lack the physical and emotional stamina of earlier years. As the relationships change, important adjustments are needed on both sides. For older people who have once enjoyed a position of authority it is never easy to step down into a subsidiary role. They can remain content only if they feel loved and appreciated and if their position and security within the family are assured. Old people need to be needed and this is easier if they can be of service to others. An old person who cultivates his grandchildren when they are young is likely to enjoy their company when he is old to their mutual benefit.

Failure to achieve adjustment is a potent cause of tension within the family. In his fear of losing status and authority the old person may be driven, consciously or unconsciously, to 'difficult' behaviour. He makes unreasonable demands upon his family and in this way becomes his own worst enemy. Conversely a member of the younger generation may fail to outgrow a dependent relationship with her parents and this too produces stress.

Family tensions

The tensions between an old person, who cannot accept an appropriate role, and the younger generation, who cannot make him feel valued, may make life difficult for both sides. This is especially marked when, out of a sense of duty, the 'children' have taken the old person to live with them, perhaps after an illness or bereavement. Tensions may, of course, occur between a mother and her daughter but are more likely to arise between 'in-laws'. Trouble is more likely and more destructive when there are unresolved emotional problems from earlier years.

Resentment

A situation which may have begun with the best of intentions on both sides becomes increasingly difficult when physical or mental frailty overtakes the old person. The younger generation may find that their social activities and holidays are restricted and as the burden of responsibility becomes heavier, resentment, probably at first unconscious, begins to arise.

This grows more quickly when others are involved. For example, a housewife may feel torn between her duty to her husband and children and her duty to the old person. She will feel worse if the presence of the old person puts unnatural restraints upon her children's activities and outings. A sense of injustice may assail her if she feels she is being left to manage single-handed while other relatives opt out. She may have anxieties about her own health or ability to cope, especially if she is getting broken nights. She may secretly be terrified of old age. Eventually, as resentment and tension grow, the stage may be set for the one thing above all which the old person wishes to avoid, his rejection by the family with whom he has made his home.

Rejection

Matters usually come to a head with a crisis, an illness, the onset of incontinence, or perhaps nocturnal restlessness. Sometimes the crisis is a 'social emergency' resulting from illness in the younger relative on whom the old person has depended, or there may have been a major family quarrel. Where the old person is ill or very frail his admission to hospital is nearly always required. Once the patient is admitted the relatives may be reluctant to have him home again or they may even reject him completely. The situation engenders much emotion among all concerned. The hospital staff, including the nurse, must not appear to criticise either the patient or the relatives. With some very difficult old people it is remarkable not that the patient has been rejected, but that the family have coped for so long.

Although total rejection is rare, lesser degrees of it are not uncommon, and it is usually the result of antagonism going back for years. It is an important part of the social worker's job to assess these situations and to see what can be done for the best.

Helping the family

Most old people are no more awkward than the rest of the human race and the majority of their relations wish to do their best for them. Many an old person can be helped by skilful social work to accept his limitations. Reconciliation may then be possible, allowing him to remain with his family.

This is usually desirable on social, economic and humanitarian grounds but the relatives may need practical help and support. However it is not always advisable for the old person to live under the same roof as his younger relatives. Many people of all ages can only get on with their relations if they are not in intimate contact with them.

The difficult person

A few old people have personalities so difficult that they bring rejection upon themselves and their problems are aggravated by the mental inflexibility which accompanies old age. They may be too self-centred and demanding to be able to adapt to the needs of others. If they are too frail to live alone their care becomes a trial to those who have to undertake it. These patients are as much a source of stress in a hospital ward or old people's home as they were to their relatives and neighbours.

The relatives and the hospital

When the patient is in hospital it is important that his relatives should feel welcome in the wards. The nurse must learn that visitors are her biggest allies in the patient's care. It is important to cultivate a sense of partnership between the ward staff and the visitors. Open visiting, at one time a concession, has become as important to the hospital as it is to the relatives, and is now recognised as a vital ingredient of good care.

Unjustified complaints, which are a source of stress to all staff, may be an indication of failure to understand the problems of the relatives. The better the communication the less likely this is to happen. Some units hold regular relatives' conferences to increase mutual understanding.

An information leaflet for visitors helps to explain the aims of treatment, the organisation of the unit and the ways in which the relations can take part in the patient's care. The Appendix gives the leaflet currently in use in Hastings.

Problems of carers

Severely disabled old people, especially the mentally infirm, can make many demands, physical, financial and emotional, on those who care for them. Although a typical carer is a woman in her mid-50s, some carers are men and many carers may be elderly, in poor health, preoccupied with other responsibilities or fearful that the burden may become too much for them psychologically or economically. Having a relative at home may add 25 per cent to a family's heating costs.

As more has to be done for the old person, the carer is less able to leave him to go to work or to follow any of her normal social activities. She suffers financially and becomes progressively isolated. Even when there are several members of a family who might help the main burden is almost always borne by one. The carer, often a daughter on her own, may feel put upon by the others. This may lead to bitterness and resentment especially if family relationships have always been stressful.

The nurse, because she knows her patients better than the other members of the hospital team and meets the visitors more often, is likely to be the first person to observe these problems in the ward.

Support for the carers

The greatest support for the carers is usually the knowledge that their efforts are recognised and appreciated. If a feeling of partnership can be developed it will be easier for them to accept help. Domiciliary nursing, services such as home help and meals-on-wheels, aids and adaptations at home, may all be needed. Day care, respite care and the assurance that readmission will be available if the patient's condition worsens, will all sustain morale. A few terminally ill patients may need the advice and support of the symptom control team and perhaps admission to a hospice, if one is available locally.

Self-help groups

Patients and their carers often benefit from meeting others with similar problems. Stroke clubs have been started in some areas and most towns have clubs for the disabled, the blind and the hard of hearing. Day Centres often run support groups for relatives. National organisations such as the Parkinson's Disease Society, the Arthritis and Rheumatism Council and the Multiple Sclerosis Society may have local branches which help the carers as much as the patients. The Association of Carers and the National Council for Carers and their Elderly Dependants (previously the National Council for the Single Woman and her Dependants) provide information and advice which help to combat isolation and loneliness.

Abuse, neglect and battering

Non-accidental injury, first recognised in children in the 1960s as 'baby battering', can occur in the elderly. As with children, the old person may be intensely loyal to the person who has assaulted him, and it is difficult to get at the truth.

Head injuries and fractures will need admission to hospital, but lesser degrees of injury may be found, especially bruising of the face, wrists or genitals for which no satisfactory explanation can be given. More commonly, rough handling, shaking, verbal abuse and threats may create a climate of intimidation and rejection. Denial of food and drink, sometimes in an attempt to reduce incontinence, over-sedation, perhaps so that the carer can obtain some sleep, or withholding prescribed drugs, can also occur. The old person may be left alone for long periods, perhaps locked in his room without adequate warmth or in wet clothing.

Financial abuse

Another category of abuse occurs when a frail old person is persuaded to hand over his money or property in exchange for provision of care. The carer is then in a position of power and may abuse his trust. Some old people give away their assets in order to claim Supplementary Benefit (Income Support) or to reduce the amount they will be required to pay for their maintenance in a local authority residential home.

Who abuses the old?

Any carer can be driven to the limit of his endurance. Incontinence and incessant purposeless activity are especially wearing. The problems will be exacerbated if the family is socially isolated, lives in poor accommodation and does not have adequate community support. Some people have a low tolerance of frustration. Danger signs are evidence of mental handicap or a history of mental illness or alcoholism in the carer. There is some evidence that battered wives may become battered grannies, probably because their children have been brought up in a climate of violence. Sometimes couples are abusive to each other all their married lives but only in old age or illness do the neighbours or authorities become involved.

The social worker will try to work out with the patient and his carers the best – or perhaps the least bad – way of providing the care he needs. However, at no time should a patient be sent home to an unwilling or hostile family unless the old person fully understands the situation and insists on returning there. Even if the patient has a legal right to return to his home, it is seldom wise to exercise it unless steps can be taken to ensure his protection and care.

For further reading:

ASSOCIATION OF CARERS. 1984. *Help at Hand: The Who, How and Where of Caring*. Association of Carers.

DARTINGTON, T. 1980. *Family Care of Old People*. London: Souvenir Press.

EASTWOOD, M. 1984. *Old Age Abuse*. Age Concern England.

GRAY, J. M. & MCKENZIE, H. 1980. *Take Care of Your Elderly Relative*. London: Allen and Unwin.

MACE, N. L., RABINS, P. V., CASTLETON, B., CLOKE, C. & McEWEN, E. 1985. *The 36-Hour Day*. Sevenoaks: Hodder and Stoughton.

6
Residential Care

It is not always possible for an old person in need of care to live with his family. There may be no close relatives, tensions within the family may be too great, or the old person may not wish to be a 'burden'. Well-disposed relatives may be unable to help because they live abroad, for example, or have other commitments which prevent them giving either the accommodation or the care that is needed. Occasionally the old person may be estranged from his descendants, usually because of troubles that go back to childhood. A father who deserted his young family or a single mother who was unable to bring up her children is not likely to receive much help from them in old age. Child abuse and alcoholism are sometimes factors too.

Under circumstances such as these, the old person has to look elsewhere should illness, infirmity or a social disaster compel him to give up living alone. A solution to this problem is likely to be provided by residential care in a nursing home or an old people's home. The need for residential care increases with age. Only 2 per cent of 75 year olds are in any kind of institutional care but at 85 the figure rises to 19 per cent.

Nursing homes

By law nursing homes have to be registered with the Health Authorities whose nursing officers inspect them regularly. Nursing homes are required to have a state registered nurse available at all times. Many homes are owned by private individuals or companies, others by charitable organisations. Some nursing homes offer a high standard of accommodation and care but the quality varies. This is partly a question of cost. Single rooms, day space, modern equipment, good food and adequate day and night staff are inevitably expensive. There are currently about 20 000 beds in private nursing homes.

Old People's Homes

Old people's homes give care and attention to the elderly and nearly 200 000 live in them. The age at entry is usually over 80 and many of the residents are very frail. The majority of homes are run by social services departments. Others are owned by voluntary societies or by private individuals. Voluntary and private homes are very unevenly distributed. In some parts of the country, particularly in the south, there are many. Elsewhere there are none.

Local Authority homes

Every local authority has a statutory duty to provide residential accommodation for persons who 'by reason of age or infirmity are in need of care and attention which is not otherwise available to them'. This duty is laid down in Part III of the National Assistance Act (1948) and for this reason these homes are sometimes spoken of as Part III accommodation. Two-thirds of the places available for old people in Great Britain are in homes of this type. In the last twenty years their numbers have expanded and an increasing proportion offer a high standard of accommodation.

The need for old people's homes depends on the availability of other services. The current trend is to develop these rather than to build more homes and indeed some homes have been closed in the last few years. Where sheltered housing, day care and domiciliary services are well developed fewer old people need to live in homes. Those that do, however, will be very frail. At least a third will have poor hearing and sight, and a tendency to incontinence. Some surveys have shown that half the residents of old people's homes are mentally impaired and there are many more such people in Part III accommodation than in mental hospitals. The majority of residents will need walking aids or wheelchairs. Two-thirds may need help at night. Local authority homes tend to be large, often with as many as fifty places. They have to take people from widely different backgrounds, solely on the basis of need. Compatibility of residents cannot be one of their primary concerns and prospective applicants rarely have much opportunity to choose their home. In most of the local authority homes bedrooms are shared except in the newest where there are more single rooms.

Voluntary Homes

Voluntary societies provide about one-fifth of the places available in old people's homes. Such homes often cater for particular groups of people, for example, clergy and their widows or ex-servicemen. Others accept only 'distressed gentlefolk' or the residents of a particular district or members of a religious faith. Still others care for old people with certain handicaps, for example, the blind.

The bodies which run these homes are numerous. Many are religious, for example the Methodist Church, convents (both Roman Catholic and Anglican), the Salvation Army and various Jewish organisations. Others are secular like the British Red Cross Society, The Women's Royal Voluntary Service, the British Legion, trade unions and charitable trusts. Many of the buildings started life as hotels or private houses to which extensions have been added, but the newer ones are often purpose-built. There are more single or double rooms than in most local authority homes. Voluntary homes can select their residents and if a person proves unsuitable he can be asked to leave.

Private Homes

Private old people's homes now provide about one-fifth of available places, a proportion which has doubled in the last ten years and will continue to rise. More people, particularly with the aid of the Attendance Allowance (see p. 28) can afford private fees and cuts in public expenditure are making it impossible for the local authorities to cope with the growing numbers of frail old people. Such money as they now have is tending to go into the provision of domiciliary services for the elderly.

Private homes have to be registered by the social services department of the local authority and they are inspected regularly. Private homes are usually small and this can give them a more homely atmosphere. Moreover in areas where there are many private homes there is a healthy element of competition which allows the old person more choice.

There are wide variations in cost according to the staff and facilities provided. Some are little more than guest houses. Others employ trained staff and are able to give their residents a good deal of care. In homes which are lightly staffed difficulties sometimes arise if a resident needs more attention than they can provide. Should he become ill he may have to move to a hospital or nursing home.

Choice of Home

There are many factors governing the choice of home for an individual patient. The most obvious is the availability of a suitable home in the area where the old person wishes to live. Some people will choose a home run for their own professional, religious or social group, even if this means moving away from their home town. For others the most important factor will be a single room, to bring their own furniture with them or to be accompanied by a pet. The patient's choice is also limited by his physical condition and the amount of care he needs. For example, a home with many stairs, no lift and few staff is suitable only for a relatively active old person.

The patient's finances are a most important consideration. In homes run by the local authority the resident pays an amount which is assessed according to his means, the balance being met from public funds. An old person entering a private home, however, is responsible for the full fees. This can lead to difficulties, especially if the patient is mentally frail, financially irresponsible, or has no relative to look after his interests. Such patients are vulnerable to exploitation and need protection.

Financial protection

For many patients the best protection is to live in a local authority home, their money being handled by the treasurer's department.

Others, if they can understand what they are doing, may be willing to give a Power of Attorney to a relative or to their solicitor who will then manage their affairs.

Where the patient is unable to understand what is involved, the services of the Court of Protection are available. The Court will appoint a responsible person to act as Receiver, and to administer the patient's finances under its direction. If there is no suitable person to act in this way the patient's affairs can be managed by the Official Solicitor.

Going into a Home

Entering a home is a major upheaval in the life of the older patient. It is a time when he needs special support and understanding. Many old people in hospital will be going into a home for the first time when they are discharged.

Such a patient may well feel anxious and insecure, and he needs time to make up his mind. If he is to settle happily in the home chosen it is important that he should feel that the decision to enter it has been his alone and that he has not been rushed into it by well-meaning friends or hospital staff. This is one of the many reasons why his previous home should never be given up until he is established in his new way of life. On the other hand he should not be allowed to live from day to day in the shelter of the hospital ward without giving thought to the morrow. It will help him to face the future realistically if he is encouraged to talk about his problems.

Living in a Home

Life in a home is bound to be very different for the old person from life in his own household. If he lived alone before, he had no one but himself to consider. If he lived with relatives, he was a member of a small group bound together by family loyalties. In a home on the other hand the old person must sacrifice some privacy and conform to the needs of the group with whom he lives. This is never easy, but it is made less difficult if the home has a stable, tolerant and permissive atmosphere, giving him a feeling of welcome and a sense of belonging.

In addition old people need to feel that as far as possible they participate in the running of the home. Sometimes a residents' committee may be appropriate but if the old people are too infirm for this they should at least be consulted on the day-to-day routine. As much choice as possible should be left to the residents. When to get up or go to bed, how to dress or what to eat become even more important in old age. Activities within the home are needed. Opportunities for hobbies, crafts, outings and even keep-fit classes may be enjoyed.

In a growing number of homes the accommodation is divided into self-contained units for six to eight residents.

Group living

Many larger homes have introduced a system of group living. No one can relate to perhaps fifty other residents and almost as many staff. If the home is divided into units of six to eight people, then each group can have its own sitting/dining area, kitchen, bathroom and bedroom. Residents are then able to make friends with each other and to maintain as much independence and self-sufficiency as possible. The staff adopt a supportive rather than a caring role.

Key worker

When the home is unsuitable for group living an alternative way to sustain individuality is for each resident to relate to a key worker. This is a care assistant assigned to each new resident with special responsibilities for his welfare and happiness. The key worker gets to know her residents and their families and makes sure that the needs of the undemanding person are not overlooked. The key worker arrangement also benefits the staff, increasing their commitment and providing greater job satisfaction.

The officer-in-charge

The quality of life in a home for both residents and staff depends primarily on the officer-in-charge.

In addition to her administrative duties her most important responsibility is to give her residents what so many have lost and others perhaps have never known, a sense that someone is concerned for their wellbeing. The elderly resident's emotional security depends on a background of affection and a sense of being valued for himself. To supply this need requires compassion, understanding, professional competence and management skill. The officer-in-charge must be able to lead her staff, select the right key workers, inspire confidence in the relatives and the committee or officials responsible for the home. All this is not easy and the job of the officer-in-charge is exacting. Her success is the key to the atmosphere in any home.

Future trends in residential care

Residential care is very expensive and for most people would not be their chosen way of life. The use of homes is changing in an effort to ensure that they are used in the most effective way and that people move into them only after alternatives have been carefully explored.

Allocation committee

The allocation committee is a good way to achieve this. Social workers from the hospital and the community meet regularly with the residential home staff to discuss proposed admissions, to make sure that every alternative has been considered, and to match clients to available vacancies. Social workers who have arranged emergency admissions in response to a domestic crisis are required to report on the situation and to consider plans for the resident's future care.

It is important for the officer-in-charge to visit the prospective resident in his own home or hospital and to provide him with an opportunity to visit before he is admitted. All this takes time and effort but it is an essential element in proper care.

Review

It is not enough, however, to make careful arrangements for admission to a home. It is important also to review the resident's progress. After a month or six weeks a 'Case Review' is held at the home between the resident, his family, the social worker who arranged his admission and the staff. If his health and circumstances have improved the resident may be able to return home. If however this is not possible and he continues to need care, he should be encouraged to bring in his personal belongings and perhaps some of his furniture to make his room as homely as possible. Until this has been done his former place of residence should not be given up.

Joint services

Residential care is no longer seen in isolation but as part of a continuum of services. The trend is towards greater flexibility by the provision of residential care, a day centre, and sheltered housing all on the same site, planned and financed jointly by the Housing and Social Services Departments with shared staff and facilities.

Such an arrangement enables an old person to move easily from one kind of care to another. For example a person who lives at home but attends the day centre may move into residential care while his daughter has a holiday and continue to attend the day centre. A resident in the home may improve enough to move to one of the flats in the sheltered housing complex. Conversely the disabled survivor of a married couple who lived together in sheltered housing may need to move into residential care after bereavement.

The mentally infirm resident

An unresolved problem is the best way to care for the mentally infirm resident. A person whose behaviour is disturbed, who gets into the wrong bed and constantly takes other people's belongings, will disrupt the lives of the other residents. Should there be, therefore, more homes specialising in the care of the mentally infirm? Or should existing homes expect to take all comers, perhaps with a special unit within the home, to cater for the needs of the more disturbed? In practice most old people's homes' residents have some degree of mental impairment but only a small proportion exhibit behaviour problems distressing to other residents.

Foster homes

As an alternative to the residential home, attempts have been made to place old people with private families. This can be a happy solution to some people's problems, especially those afflicted by loneliness rather than physical frailty. The very frail usually require more attention than can reasonably be expected in a foster home.

For further reading:

AVEBURY, K. 1984. *Home Life: A code of practice for residential care.* Report of a working party sponsored by D. H. S. S. Centre for Policy on Ageing.

BREARLEY, C. P. 1977. *Residential Work with the Elderly.* London: Routledge and Kegan Paul.

DHSS. 1980. *Growing Old in Brighton.* HMSO.

NORMAN, A. J. 1984. *Bricks and Mortals.* Centre for Policy on Ageing.

7
The Department of Medicine for the Elderly (Organisation – Assessment – Nursing Process)

Old people are the principal users of most departments of the hospital, but this chapter will concentrate on the department specifically intended for the older patient, the geriatric unit.

Regrettably the scientific word geriatric has entered common speech in a way that emphasises the negative aspect of old age. Patients and their relatives are therefore sometimes unhappy at the thought of treatment in such a department. It may be better to speak of a Department of Geriatric Medicine, but perhaps best of all from the point of view of public relations, is to speak of the Department of Medicine for the Elderly. This is the title which was adopted in Hastings in 1981.

A specialist unit is necessary because the elderly and their relatives require a medical department where they will be welcomed and not treated as a nuisance or as potential bed blockers. The elderly have multiple illnesses, mental factors are common, physical disability is very important and social problems almost universal. A multidisciplinary team approach is essential if their numerous problems are to be solved.

It is vital that the department should be based in a district general hospital with access to full facilities for investigation and treatment. Some units specialise in the treatment of patients with a particular need for their facilities. Others take in addition all patients from the district over a certain age. Often this is 75.

Physical illness

An acute physical illness or an acute exacerbation of a chronic illness is the main reason for admission to hospital. A fall is the commonest single presentation of illness in the elderly but there are numerous possible reasons for the fall which require investigation and treatment.

Mental illness

In the older patient physical and mental illness are closely inter-
woven but it is usually clear which is the most important. In
some cases, however, there is doubt. An assessment ward jointly
staffed by a psychiatrist and a physician specialising in the care of the
elderly can then be of value. After a period of observation and
investigation the patient is transferred by agreement to the
appropriate department for further treatment if he cannot go home.

Social problems

Social factors are as important as medical ones in the decision to
send a patient to hospital. For example a person who lives alone is
more likely to be admitted than someone with a family to look after
him. Moreover an old person who is disabled but not acutely ill may
require admission as a social emergency if he is suddenly deprived of
the services of his principal helper. Or a period in hospital may be
arranged after consultation with the social worker, to enable the
patient's relative to have a holiday. Sometimes regular intermittent
admissions help the family to share with the hospital the burden of
his care.

Rehabilitation

The department must provide good facilities for rehabilitation of
the older patient. An atmosphere of rehabilitation is the hallmark of
every good unit (see Chapter 9).

Discharge

In a well run department every effort will be made to achieve
early discharge. Only in this way will it be possible to provide a bed
for the next person urgently needing admission. Younger patients
can usually return home as soon as their medical condition allows.
The older patient's discharge has to be specially prepared. The
relatives as well as the patient must be consulted and suitable
arrangements made with the general practitioner team and the social
services.

Successful discharge is only possible if the necessary community
services are available. If home help for example, or a place in an old
people's home cannot be provided the patient may have to wait in
hospital. This is bad for his morale and for the efficiency of the

hospital. Hospital and community services are interdependent and the patient suffers if either is inadequate.

Continuing care

For the few patients who cannot be discharged, including some who are dying, the department must provide continuing care and treatment. At this stage the older patient is not always suitably placed in the district general hospital. A smaller unit nearer his home may meet his needs better.

Outpatient care

Most people prefer to be treated at home. Where circumstances allow, the patient may attend the geriatric outpatient clinic or day hospital. If necessary the general practitioner can arrange for a domiciliary consultation with the physician in geriatric medicine at the patient's home.

Teaching and research

The department should be a centre of teaching and research. In this way it creates interest in the problems of the older patient and raises the standard of his care.

Progressive patient care

The complex functions of the department are reflected in its structure. Most units consist of a series of different wards, each with its special purpose. The patient moves from one part of the unit to another as his needs in treatment change. He may move within the ward if it is suitably organised or he may be transferred from one ward to another. This system is known as progressive patient care. A new patient goes first to an acute unit for assessment and immediate treatment. Once the acute phase is over his needs change. The requirement then is for rehabilitation or continued nursing care. If he has found his feet, a short period in a ward for ambulant patients helps consolidate recovery. If full independence is necessary before discharge a self-care unit will help to achieve it.

An alternative to progressive patient care practised in some units is to provide all phases of care including long-stay in one ward. Special efforts can then be made to bring the patient back to the ward where he is already known should he require readmission. This very humane policy is only possible when every ward in the department can function as an acute ward in a district general hospital with full facilities for investigation. Only one or two departments, notably Hull, are blessed with these advantages.

Assessment

When a patient comes to hospital he needs assessment. This involves more than merely attaching names to his diseases. It implies an attempt to comprehend all his problems as fully as possible. The first medical assessment is made on the patient's admission but it will be reviewed on every ward round. Assessment has three aspects, medical, functional and social. The nursing assessment will be considered later.

Medical assessment

The hospital doctor will try to define the most pressing medical need and to write a medical problem list. Assisted by the letter from the general practitioner he will attempt to take a history. The patient may be able to give a good account, but he may be confused, forgetful or even unconscious. It is always helpful to check his story and to fill out the details by talking to any relative, friend or neighbour who may have accompanied him to hospital or who visits him later. The nurse can often help in this.

The doctor's examination will be as complete as he can make it. In addition to checking the heart, chest, abdomen and nervous system the doctor will look for pressure sores and will pay special attention to the joints, feet, eyes and ears. A rectal examination is essential and, of course, a urine test. The examination will be supplemented by a number of routine investigations. These will include a full blood count to exclude anaemia, a blood sugar to exclude diabetes, an estimation of urea and electrolytes as tests of kidney function and a number of other tests to check liver function, alkaline phosphatase, renal function, calcium and protein levels. In many units routine thyroid function tests are performed also. A chest X-ray and an electrocardiogram are likely to be routine investigations. Other tests may be ordered as needed.

Mental scoring

An important part of medical assessment is to look for mental impairment which may be present in up to half of those admitted to a geriatric unit. Mental impairment is likely to be suspected if the nurse or doctor finds it difficult to get a clear history from the patient. Sometimes however the patient appears to give a good history which, when it is checked, proves to be largely fanciful. So it is useful to quantify the patient's mental function by the routine use of a mental score.

There are many mental scoring systems now available and all are probably of equal usefulness. In Hastings the ten point mental status questionnaire (MSQ) is used. This test, devised by Dr Alvin Goldfarb of New York and introduced into this country by Dr L. A. Wilson, gives a rapid guide to the patient's mental capacity and correlates well with his performance in the activities of living.

Mental status questionnaire
  1 What is this town?
  2 What month were you born?
  3 What is this place?
  4 What is your age?
  5 What month is it now?
  6 What year were you born?
  7 Who is the Prime Minister?
  8 What year is it now?
  9 What is the date today?
 10 Who was the last Prime Minister?

One point is given for each correct answer and a normal old person gets 9 or 10. Moderately impaired patients score between 6 and 8 but a patient with severe brain failure scores 5 or less. When a patient has a low score at first testing and does better on a later occasion, this usually indicates the clearing of a temporary incident of acute brain failure.

The test is unreliable if the patient cannot speak clearly because of dysphasia, if he is deaf, or if he does not understand the English language. Patients who are deeply depressed may not be able to make the effort to answer the questions. The same is true of patients who are under sedation.

The MSQ should certainly be done during the patient's first day or two in hospital, but it is often wise to postpone it until he has had a chance to settle in.

Functional assessment

Functional assessment is a common sense way of looking at the patient. What the whole team needs to know is an answer to the question, 'What can he do?' Can he transfer from bed to chair? Can he get out of this chair and walk to the toilet? How much assistance is required? Can he wash and dress himself? Is he continent, completely or only with assistance from the nurses? Can he do stairs? Can he make a cup of tea, cook a meal and wash up? What is his mental state? How is his memory?

It is possible to ask a wide range of questions seeking a detailed assessment, so many in fact that it is hard to remember all of them. In practice the four key questions concern continence, mobility, mental state and the ability to dress.

A useful reminder, invented by Dr P. S. Bhatia, is to think of the word CARD. C reminds us to ask about continence and bladder function; A stands for ambulant and reminds us to ask about mobility and the help required to achieve it; R stands for rational to which state the mental score is a useful pointer; D stands for dressing, a complex activity exercising both mind and body. Those who can dress themselves unaided usually do well.

Others may prefer to think of the 3 Ms, invented by Dr William Fine. The 3 Ms stand for mobility, micturition and mental function.

Members of each profession, the doctor, the nurse, the physiotherapist, the occupational therapist and the social worker tend to see the patient in different ways. An agreed system helps to provide a common framework when together they assess his function.

The importance of functional assessment increases when the patient is over the acute stage of his illness. In the end it is what he can do for himself which determines when he can leave hospital.

Social assessment

A proper assessment of the older patient cannot be made without a knowledge of his social circumstances. This information may be obtained by the social worker, doctor, nurse or health visitor at a domiciliary visit before admission or in hospital if the patient has been admitted as an emergency.

It is necessary to establish where and how the patient lives, as is now done in the nursing process. For example, an old man living with a devoted, healthy and much younger wife in a convenient modern bungalow is likely to be able to go home in spite of considerable disability. An identical illness in an elderly widow living alone in a top floor bed-sitting room with a lavatory two flights of stairs away will totally prevent her returning to her former way of life and the help of the social worker will be essential.

The social worker is the hospital's link with the community. She will need to get to know the patient and determine his reaction to illness. Adjustment to disability is vital to successful rehabilitation. A highly skilled activity of the social worker is to help the patient come to terms with his situation and make realistic plans for the future, a process which inevitably takes time. It may be necessary also for her to interpret the patient's needs and wishes to other members of the team and to the relatives.

The social worker will need to know also how the relatives feel. They may have a sense of guilt or other anxiety. Their problems may be no less pressing than those of the patient. All this must be understood before the social worker can help them come to terms with the situation. It is part of her responsibility then to interpret, within the bounds of confidentiality, this information to the other members of staff so that they too may be more tolerant and understanding.

Finally she must preserve the patient's place in the community by ensuring that his home is kept for him until he is ready to return to it or until alternative plans have been made.

When the time comes for his discharge she must arrange also his support at home.

Nursing assessment

The doctor's assessment leads to decisions about immediate medical treatment. Equally important is the plan for the patient's nursing care. This is based on the principles of the nursing process which is well suited to the needs of the older patient.

The nursing process

The first step is to take a nursing history. Although this will to some extent overlap with the medical history its purposes and emphasis are different. The aims are to get to know the patient as an individual, to understand his illness and to ascertain his problems and anxieties. In this way the nurse can begin to plan the way to meet his needs. This is the foundation of good care.

In the assessment of the older patient it is important for the nurse to appreciate that the relatives also may have their problems and these too must be understood.

Nursing history

The form of the nursing history differs in various departments but the main points are common to all.

As well as the personal details the nurse will ask about eating and drinking habits, patterns of sleep, bowel and bladder function, washing, dressing and other activities of living. She will also want to know whether the patient uses spectacles, dentures or a hearing aid and, if so, whether he has them with him. She will try and find out what understanding the patient and his relatives have of his illness and his treatment.

For the care of the older patient some social information, too, is vital. His housing, the way he has been living, the support he has had from family and friends, the help he has been receiving from the domiciliary services will all need to be recorded. This may reveal a need to involve the social worker at an early stage.

There is inevitably some overlap with the social assessment as there is with the medical. All this information is unlikely to be obtainable immediately, especially if the patient has been admitted as an emergency. The picture is likely to be built up gradually over several days. Although it is always right to give full weight to the patient's account it is also necessary to consult with those who care for him at home.

There is a tension between collecting information which may be vital for the understanding of the patient's needs and the maintenance of confidentiality. The nurse needs to be aware of these problems which are inseparable from the nursing process.

For further reading:

COAKLEY, D. (Ed). 1982. *Establishing a Geriatric Service*. Beckenham: Croom Helm.

GARRETT, G. 1983. *Health Needs of the Elderly*. London: Macmillan.

GRAHAM, J. M. & HODKINSON, H. M. 1983. *Effective Geriatric Medicine*. HMSO.

KRATZ, C. R. (Ed). 1980. *The Nursing Process*. Eastbourne: Baillière Tindall.

8
Care in Different Wards

Under a system of progressive patient care each ward has its own purpose, emphasising a different aspect of treatment according to the patient's changing needs.

Acute unit

The acute unit receives all new patients and the emphasis is on medical assessment and the treatment of acute illness. There will be a number of deaths, perhaps one in four of all those admitted. The usual length of stay is about ten days, but if a patient requires prolonged investigation, intensive medical treatment or special nursing, he can be kept in the acute unit for as long as is necessary.

Acute wards for the elderly, like all other acute wards, are very busy and have a high turnover. They must therefore be well staffed with a high proportion of trained nurses. There are many enquiries from relatives and a great deal of telephoning and paper work for which a ward clerk is indispensable.

About half the patients will be heavily dependent. They may be unconscious or require intravenous treatment or other specialised care. It is important to identify the patients who are at risk for pressure sores in order that preventive measures may be taken. This may be done by immediate clinical assessment, those who are most ill, dehydrated, wasted or immobile being at greatest risk.

The risk may be quantified by means of the Norton score. The patient is 'scored' by considering his physical condition, his mental state, his activity, his mobility in bed or chair and his degree of continence. He is given a mark from 1 − 4 for each of these features, a high mark indicating a low risk of pressure sores and a low mark a high risk (Fig. 2). A score of 14 or less indicates that the patient is at some risk of developing pressure sores. The patient should be re-scored at intervals and his nursing care reviewed.

Transfers from ward to ward

The older patient may not expect to be moved from the acute ward and it is important to prepare him psychologically. He must be

A. Physical Condition		B. Mental Condition		C. Activity		D. Mobility		E. Incontinent	
Good	4	Alert	4	Ambulant	4	Full	4	Not	4
Fair	3	Apathetic	3	Walk/help	3	Slightly limited	3	Occasionally	3
Poor	2	Confused	2	Chairbound	2	Very limited	2	Usually/urine	2
Very bad	1	Stuporous	1	Bedfast	1	Immobile	1	Doubly	1

Instructions for use:
(1) Assess the patient's condition and score accordingly (1–4) under each heading (A to E).
(2) Total the scores together.
(3) A total of 14 and below indicates a patient is at risk and preventive measures should be taken. The lower the total, the higher the risk.
(4) Assess the patient regularly.

Source: Norton *et al.* (1975).

Fig. 2 The Norton scoring system

helped to feel that each move is a planned step forward. The procedure is explained on admission, and as the patient is likely to be forgetful, every opportunity must be taken to remind him and his relatives. It is an advantage if the nurse in charge of the ward to which he is going can meet him before he moves. When he arrives in the new ward he must be welcomed and introduced to the other patients. The toilet arrangements must be explained to him and he must be shown his bedroom and the layout of the ward.

Continuity of nursing information is provided by the patient's nursing notes which, with his medical notes, accompany him wherever he goes.

The relatives, too, must be kept in the picture. They need as much information as possible. They may find the hospital unfamiliar and frightening. They should be given an explanatory leaflet (see Appendix) and informed whenever the patient is to be moved. They need as much contact with the nursing and medical staff as possible and any offer to help with the patient's care, for example in feeding, should be encouraged. Open visiting multiplies the opportunities for communication and it is often helpful if the relatives can be present when the doctor is doing his round. At all times the relatives must be made welcome. They should never be made to feel intruders.

Rehabilitation unit

A special feature of any Department of Medicine for the Elderly is the way in which a rehabilitative approach is part and parcel of the patient's care from the moment he comes into hospital. Many patients go home directly from the acute ward but there are others for whom recovery is difficult and prolonged. For them a rehabilitation unit is an indispensable element in progressive patient care. The unit may comprise a series of wards for patients at different stages of recovery or there may be mixed rehabilitation wards which take people with varying degrees of disability.

The primary task of the rehabilitation unit is to get the patient on his feet again. Most will be convalescent and the nurse must use all her skill to help the patient help himself. An encouraging atmosphere is important. The old person must feel accepted as an individual with a sense that his needs are understood. Under these conditions most patients recover their self-confidence and co-operate in their reablement.

Ward arrangements for rehabilitation

Rehabilitation requires plenty of day space, about 6 sq m for every patient in the ward. Patients should sit in small groups, preferably round a table for conversation, games and diversional activities. The dining area should be separate from the sitting area to encourage movement and provide a change of scene. Lavatories, one to every four patients, must be near at hand. No patient should be further than 10 m (33 ft) from a lavatory at any time. There must be adequate storage space for physiotherapy and occupational therapy equipment.

The bed area must be equipped with suitable furniture, including adjustable height beds, grab chains and wardrobe lockers. The St. Helen's Hospital locker is suitable for this purpose (see Fig. 33a). A few chairs should be mobile so that a patient who cannot walk may readily be moved from bedside to day room. Every patient should have a commode by his bed at night. A suitable model can double as a bedside chair by day. Privacy must be assured by individual bed curtaining.

The ambulant unit

Some units have special wards for patients who can walk. The patient should normally be up and dressed all day and spend his time in the day room, with perhaps an afternoon rest on his bed. Such a ward can be fairly lightly staffed, and should be equipped with low beds so that the patient can easily get in and out. Should he become ill, however, he will need to be moved out of the ambulant ward, which is neither staffed nor equipped to deal with emergencies. The ambulant ward should give the patients plenty of practice in the activities of living. Occupational therapy is directed towards the re-establishment of personal and domestic skills. Group exercises, perhaps to music, are useful. It is often important that the patient should practice climbing stairs.

Self-care unit

The self-care unit caters for those who need practice in caring for themselves before they are discharged. It should have single bedrooms if possible and its own bathroom, toilet, sitting room and kitchen where patients can prepare their meals under the supervision of the occupational therapist. The therapist not only observes the patient in the kitchen but, in consultation with the nurse, evaluates his need for help in the activities of living. The self-care unit thus provides an ideal means of functional assessment.

The self-care unit may include an AL flat where the patient who is to live alone after discharge may try himself out. The flat may also be used to help an able bodied relative to learn to care for a handicapped member of the family. In this way the patient and his relatives gain confidence that they will be able to manage at home with domiciliary support if required.

Case conference

As at every other stage of his treatment, the patient in the ambulant or self-care unit needs regular assessment. At this stage the functional and social aspects are often of greater importance than the medical and it is particularly important for the doctor, the social worker, the remedial therapist and the nurses to keep in close touch, not only with each other but with the community health and social services. Communication is best achieved by a regular case conference. An important function of the case conference is to guide all concerned in the patient's rehabilitation programme and the policy for his future management. So many people are involved, both in the hospital and in the community, that it is vital for them to meet. They thus learn to value each other's professional contribution and the pooling of information enables realistic plans to be made for the patient's future.

Communication

When the patient is discharged it is vital that the information about him should be communicated speedily to his general practitioner and to the community nurses. The Department of Medicine for the Elderly should have an efficient secretarial service so that a discharge letter can be dictated, typed, signed and posted to the general practitioner the day the patient leaves hospital. In addition a continuity of patient care form, completed by the ward sister, should go to the Primary Health Care Team on the day he leaves hospital, or accompany him if he moves to a nursing home or residential care (Fig. 3).

Aftercare

Many old people need continued medical and social supervision after their discharge from hospital. The responsibility for this falls primarily upon the general practitioner but he may be glad of help from the hospital's follow-up clinic. In some places a Liaison Health Visitor attached to the Department of Medicine for the Elderly visits the patient within 48 hours of discharge. This enables her to check that the patient and his family understand his medication and that the plans for his support in the community are working as arranged.

Day Hospital

An important element contributing to the support of the elderly in the community is the day hospital. It provides facilities for medical assessment, investigation and rehabilitation for patients who are able to live at home.

Up to half of those attending a day hospital will be coming for continued rehabilitation and support after discharge from the ward. The remainder will have been referred by a general practitioner for rehabilitation. Most will have difficulty in walking due to stroke, Parkinson's disease, cervical myelopathy or other neurological troubles. Some also will have mental impairment.

It is important to define the reason for the patient's attendance at the day hospital and the aims of treatment. This will be decided by the doctor in consultation with other members of the multidisciplinary team. Treatment offered in a day hospital may include physiotherapy for walking and balance, occupational therapy training in the activities of living, speech therapy, observation of the patient's behaviour and response to drugs or a chance to consult with the social worker. The nurse may be able to give advice about such problems as constipation, the management of incontinence and nutrition. The day hospital provides a good opportunity to try out various aids and gadgets and wheelchair clinics may be held.

The day hospital also contributes to the support of the family. The staff can advise and teach relatives about ways to help the patient. Relatives are welcome to visit the day hospital and once they have met the staff are often glad to seek advice by telephone. The day hospital also provides a point of contact with community services. Sometimes the remedial therapists visit their patients at home to assess the need for adaptations to the house or furniture.

The main objective of attendance at the day hospital is to find ways of increasing the patient's independence. Most patients will come 2 or 3 times a week at first. Then the frequency of their attendance is tailed off over two or three months. If a patient attends the day hospital for too long he may become dependent upon it, the opposite of what is intended. Most day hospitals find that things go best if the patient does not attend more than 20 times in any one course of treatment. It is important that when a patient has reached his peak of independence he should be discharged. But he can always be offered further courses of treatment should the need arise.

Day centres

Patients whose needs are social rather than medical can benefit from attendance at a day centre which is usually run by the social services department or a voluntary organisation. Day centres offer transport, a range of social activities, an opportunity for craft work and meals. They also offer regular relief for the family as well as a welcome day out for the disabled old person.

In both day hospitals and day centres baths, laundry facilities, hairwashing and chiropody are usually available. Day centres, not being part of the National Health Service, usually make a small charge for attendance.

Day centres may be purpose built or held in church halls or in local authority homes. They may provide a valuable means of support to those who have completed a period of treatment in a day hospital.

Continuing care

Some patients, usually because of mental impairment added to gross physical handicap, fail to achieve rehabilitation. It becomes apparent that they will not regain their independence.

HASTINGS HEALTH AUTHORITY

CONTINUITY OF CARE

Unit No. ....

FROM: Hospital.................

Ward.................

TO: ....

Surname.................   Forenames ....   Mr./Mrs./Miss
                                                                                       Widower/Widow

Address.................

....   Tel. No. ....

D.O.B. ....   G.P. ....   Community Sister/H.V.:—

Next of Kin ....   Relationship. ....

Address. ....   Tel. No. ....   Tel. No. ....

HOSPITAL/COMMUNITY/CARE *(Delete as Necessary)*

Date Admitted. ....   Date Discharged/Transferred. ....   T ....

Diagnosis. ....   Operation &/or Treatment Given:—   P ....

Diet. ....   R ....

Treatment required ....   B.P. ....

....

....   Transport Necessary   YES/NO

Drugs prescribed to take home ....   Transport Arranged   YES/NO

....

....

....

Out Patient Treatment, e.g. Day Hospital, Physio., etc. ....
Out Patient Appointment. ....

PATIENT'S GENERAL CONDITION *(Please Tick)*

Mobility

1. Ambulant ☐
2. Walks with Aid (State Aid)
   ....
3. Walks with Help (No Aid) ☐
4. Up in chair ☐
5. Bedfast ☐

Mental

1. Alert
2. Slightly confused
3. Severely confused
   —Day
   —Night
   —Continually

Handicaps

1. Deaf ☐
2. Blind ☐
3. Partially Sighted
4. Arthritic ☐
5. Other (Please state) ☐
   ☐
   ....

Incontinence

1. Urine ☐
   Day/Night/Both ☐
2. Faeces— ☐
   Day/Night/Both ☐
   Pressure Areas—
   1. Healthy
   2. Unhealthy

☐☐

(Elaborate) ....

SOCIAL CONDITIONS *(Delete as Necessary)*

1. Living Alone   YES/NO
2. Help Available   YES/NO
3. Housing Facilities   ADEQUATE/INADEQUATE
   (Please elaborate if necessary)
   ....
4. Type of Home. ....

SERVICES REQUESTED *(Please Tick)*

1. Community Nursing Sister
2. Health Visitor
3. Liaison H. V./Sister
4. Social Worker
5. Home Help
6. Meals on Wheels
7. Voluntary Worker
8. P.H.I.C.S. Scheme

☐ ☐ ☐ ☐ ☐ ☐ ☐ ☐

Signed ....   Designation ....   Date. ....

Fig. 3 Continuity of care form

Some of these severely disabled patients will have relatives who can care for them at home with help from the domiciliary services and perhaps regular periods of relief at the day hospital or through respite admissions. Others may choose a nursing home. But some, usually the most dependent or those with problems of behaviour, will need transfer to the hospital's continuing care unit.

Continuing care unit

The aim of a continuing care or long-stay unit should be to preserve the older patient's individuality and to enable him to live as full a life as possible. Long-stay patients are not very numerous in relation to the total numbers admitted but because they stay so long they occupy up to half the available beds. In Hastings less than 5 per cent of patients admitted to the Department of Medicine for the Elderly require long-stay care in hospital. Three-quarters of them are likely to be women. Four out of five will die within two years.

For these patients the hospital becomes their home for the last period of their life and this must affect the way in which the nurses approach them. The priorities of the acute ward with its emphasis on treatment and cure are inappropriate. The atmosphere should be informal and permissive. The patient should feel that he is accepted, that his wishes are considered and that he has some say in what happens to him. Whether to sit in this chair or that, for example, may be a matter of great importance to a person whose freedom of choice is restricted in so many ways. In a well run continuing care ward the nurses should sit down with the patients for part of every day, conversing or playing games with them. The long-stay patient may like to be surrounded by souvenirs of his former life, and should be encouraged to display photographs of his family and home.

The daily routine of the long-stay patient is bound to follow a fairly fixed pattern, but he should have some choice about when he gets up and when he goes to bed. He should be up and dressed and the hospital should aim to have a personalised clothing system, so that he does not have to wear clothes from a common pool. Wherever possible he should spend his time in a day room. The majority of the patients will be mentally impaired, but those who are not may need to be separated. All should be encouraged to do anything they can for themselves.

Activities

The opportunity to take part in a range of activities is an important element in the life of a long-stay patient. Each ward should have a supply of board games, dominoes and cards as well as newspapers and magazines. A conversation about the weather and current events can be used to keep patients in touch with reality. There should be a reality orientation board on which is written the name of the ward, the date, a comment about the weather and perhaps the time of the next meal.

Music. There is also a place for reminiscence and discussion. Music can stir people's emotions and memories. Record programmes and sing-songs are much enjoyed. Exercises to music, including dancing, are a pleasant way to keep the joints loose and the patients mobile.

Art. Many old people have artistic and creative ability and the skilled therapist or art tutor knows how to release their talents. Some will enjoy looking at books containing reproductions of famous pictures. Others, even the most infirm, may produce paintings and handicrafts which excite admiration. To show the patient that he can still enjoy learning right at the end of his life and can contribute to society helps his morale wonderfully.

Outings. The long-stay patient can also enjoy the open air and most continuing care units have a garden where the patients can sit and sometimes raised flower beds and a greenhouse where they may work.

Outings, too, give pleasurable anticipation, are enjoyable at the time and can be talked about afterwards.

Calendar. A useful feature of a continuing care ward is a social activities calendar. A large board placed on the wall is divided into spaces for each day of the week and the social events of each day are entered in the appropriate spaces. This shows at a glance the activity of the unit. It is reassuring to patients, relatives and staff to see how much activity can go on in a well planned long-stay unit (Fig. 4).

All such activities raise morale and help the patient to live until he dies. There are many ways to organise activities. In some units it is done by the occupational therapists and their helpers, in others by the nurses or by volunteers.

Physiotherapy

Physiotherapy plays a smaller part in the continuing care unit than in the acute and rehabilitation units. But the patient who unexpectedly begins to improve may need special attention,

WARD 3 . St. Helen's Hospital				
Programme of Activities – Week beginning 6th May 1985				
MONDAY 6th May	9 AM 10 AM 10-30 AM	DAILY PAPER COFFEE NEEDLEWORK	1-45 PM 2 PM 3 PM	KEEP FIT FLOOR GAMES TEA
TUESDAY 7th May	9 AM 10 AM 10-30 AM	DAILY PAPER COFFEE COOKERY	1-45 PM 2 PM 3 PM	KEEP FIT "TELL ME" QUIZ TEA
WEDNESDAY 8th May	9 AM 10 AM 10-30 AM	DAILY PAPER COFFEE GARDENING	1-45 PM 2 PM 3 PM	KEEP FIT TABLE GAMES TEA
THURSDAY 9th May	9 AM 10 AM 10-30 AM	DAILY PAPER COFFEE PAINTING	1-45 PM 2 PM 3 PM	KEEP FIT REALITY ORIENTATION TEA
FRIDAY 10th May	9 AM 10 AM 10-30 AM	DAILY PAPER COFFEE OUTING	1-45 PM 2 PM 3 PM	KEEP FIT BINGO TEA

Fig. 4 Activities programme

especially to strengthen his mobility. Heat or ice treatment for the relief of pain and ultraviolet light for the management of pressure sores may also be needed from time to time.

Voluntary help

Voluntary helpers have a special part to play in continuing care. They can do much to enhance the older patient's quality of life. They bring him the gift of their time and they can listen to him in a way which is seldom possible for any professional, whether nurse, therapist or doctor. Such befriending builds up the patient's confidence and reminds him that he is still a person of value. Volunteers may read to him, play games with him and help him with his letters. They may also participate in group activities, outings and entertainment.

The hospital library is usually run by volunteers from the Red Cross. The WRVS or the hospital's League of Friends may run a shop. In larger units the hospital may have a social centre where patients and visitors can meet over a cup of tea away from the ward.

The British Red Cross picture library is much appreciated. Local artists may be glad of an opportunity to exhibit in the hospital, but it is still better when the walls are decorated by the work of the patients themselves.

Good volunteers are of all ages and schoolchildren and students may bring much needed life to a ward for the elderly. Volunteers bring the local community into the hospital. When the hospital is felt to belong to those who live in the neighbourhood a positive atmosphere is easier to maintain and funds may be raised by the League of Friends to improve its amenities.

Voluntary Help Organiser

Voluntary work does, however, need to be organised and the Voluntary Help Organiser or Voluntary Services Co-ordinator is a key figure in the hospital for the elderly. Her job is to recruit suitable people and to find them appropriate tasks which they will enjoy doing and which improve the patient's quality of life. The volunteer needs to be identified by suitable clothing. In St. Helen's Hospital, Hastings, volunteers wear a red tabard or a name badge. Relationships between nurses and volunteers take a little working out. Both volunteers and professionals may feel uneasy with each other at first, but once their roles are clearly understood things will go smoothly. One of the skills of the Voluntary Help Organiser is to identify ways in which the contribution of the volunteers will assist and not hinder the nurses.

Clergy

Clergy, especially the hospital chaplains, give valuable help, not only by holding services, but by their visits and counsel. They remind the patient and those who care for him that life has a spiritual as well as a physical dimension.

Emotional problems in continuing care

The greatest emotional need of any patient in hospital, especially when he must stay a long time, is to feel that his significance as an individual is appreciated. The reader should look again at the poem at the end of Chapter 1.

The staff, too, have their emotional needs. Long-stay work is an indispensable part of the care of the elderly but it is often misunderstood and underrated. Those who work in continuing care need to feel that their contribution is valued, not only for the physical burden which the work involves but also for the skill with which they respond to the emotional needs of their patients.

The priorities of long-stay care are so different from those of the acute wards that it is difficult for nurses who have not worked in this situation to appreciate their importance. In particular the staff need support from their managers, the administration and the medical staff. If this is lacking they will in turn undervalue themselves and their patients, a process which will destroy their own job satisfaction and lead to apathy, neglect or even cruelty.

Results of continuing care

The majority of patients in a continuing care unit will be there for the remainder of their lives but they must nonetheless be constantly re-assessed. A patient may go to a continuing care ward after failing in a rehabilitation unit. Occasionally this is because he found the pressure too much for him and gave up trying. In the more relaxed atmosphere of the continuing care unit his emotional tensions subside and he begins to do better. Under these happier circumstances an unexpected improvement may set in, which will allow his discharge from hospital after all.

In a continuing care unit the patient is liable to develop new complications of his original illness or even some new disease. Thus his medical treatment must be reviewed regularly. It is particularly important that his medical prescriptions should not be unthinkingly renewed. The best long-stay units have the smallest drug bills because the patients' needs are met by better human relations and not by tranquillisers.

For further reading:

BROCKLEHURST, J. C. & TUCKER, J. S. 1980. *Progress in Geriatric Day Care*. King Edward's Hospital Fund for London.

COPP, L. A. (Ed). 1981. *Care of the Ageing*. Edinburgh: Churchill Livingstone.

DAVIES, E. M. 1984. *Let's Get Moving: Group Activation of Elderly People*. Mitcham: Age Concern.

DENHAM, M. J. (Ed). 1983. *Care of the Long Stay Elderly Patient*. Beckenham: Croom Helm.

GODLOVE, C., RICHARD, L. & RODWELL, G. 1981. *Time for Action*. University of Sheffield Printing Unit.

NORTON, D., MCLAREN, R. & EXTON-SMITH, A. N. 1976. *An Investigation of Geriatric Nursing Problems in Hospital*. Edinburgh: Churchill Livingstone.

WELLS, T. J. 1980. *Problems in Geriatric Nursing Care*. Edinburgh: Churchill Livingstone.

9
Principles of Rehabilitation

Rehabilitation is the process whereby the older patient is helped to regain the greatest possible degree of personal independence. He needs the help of a team because nurses, therapists, social workers and doctors all see him differently. It is only by combining their skills that they can meet his needs and help him to achieve the fullest degree of recovery that is possible for him.

The roles of the various members of the rehabilitation team inevitably overlap and this is as it should be. By working closely together the team generates an atmosphere of activity and optimism which is the hallmark of a good department. An understanding of rehabilitation is therefore essential for the nursing care of the older patient.

The nurse

The nurse has a key role in the rehabilitation team. Nurses are the only members of the team who treat all the patients and are available seven days a week. Even at night the nurse can contribute to the patient's rehabilitation (see p. 127).

If the staff encourage the patient to feed, wash and dress himself then he will make progress. If they insist on doing these things for him they will reinforce his dependency. If they take time to help him walk to the lavatory he will become more active and confident. It may sometimes be necessary, if the call of nature is urgent, to wheel him to the toilet quickly, but if at all possible the nurse should make sure that he walks back.

By training, experience and discussion with other members of the team the nurse learns when she must withdraw her services to help the patient help himself. Her objective, in common with other members of the team, is, as Dr T. N. Rudd puts it, to help the patient live to the hilt of his capacities.

An individual programme that will increase the patient's independence is an essential part of the nursing process (see p. 120).

The physiotherapist

The aim of the physiotherapist is to restore as far as possible the patient's mobility and function. As in the nursing process she will begin with an assessment of his disabilities and will make a plan of treatment. No one can be rehabilitated against his will and it is vital that the patient feels that his needs are understood and that he is involved in the planning.

For example a patient with a recent stroke must be positioned in ways which will subsequently favour recovery of function. A patient with a chest infection may need help to raise his sputum. A patient who has lost the power to walk may need help to find his feet again. He may need training to balance in the sitting position before he can stand. A patient with a painful joint may need ice or ultrasound before he can use it. All this may take days, weeks or months.

In all that she does the physiotherapist aims to get the patient moving, and she will work in close co-operation with the occupational therapist and other members of the team. One of the nurse's responsibilities is to keep the patient moving and ensure that he makes full use of the function he has been helped to regain.

The occupational therapist

The occupational therapist is complementary to the physiotherapist and neither can be fully effective without the other. The aim of the occupational therapist is to help the patient make use of his recovering powers in daily life, for example in dressing. She is the expert in functional assessment. She can discover what handicaps the patient in the activities of living, for example perceptual disorders in a patient with a stroke. She can help him by special training and perhaps by supplying him with aids, now happily called by Dr Heinz Wolff 'Tools for living'.

By the appropriate choice of remedial activities and by observing the patient's performance the occupational therapist can continue the work done by the physiotherapist. Once the patient can use his limbs a little he will find exercises more interesting if they are harnessed to creative activity. It is the occupational therapist's job to discover what type of activity is best suited to his disability and temperament. In her assessment and teaching of patients she will be assisted by occupational therapy helpers and perhaps by other experts, such as technical instructors and craft workers. Purposeful activities are the most suitable, for example cooking, housework, gardening, printing, woodwork and metalwork. An enjoyable occupation gives the patient encouragement and almost without his realising it helps him to regain mobility, strength and balance.

Another important aspect of the occupational therapist's work is to draw disabled patients back into the main stream of life by psychological stimulation. This she does through work performed in groups and through art, music, games and other social activities. For the patient with mental impairment she may use the technique of Reality Orientation (RO), reminding the patient repeatedly who he is, where he is, what the time is and what he will be doing next. For the demoralised patient she may use make up and manicure to rebuild self-esteem.

An expanding part of occupational therapy is the pre-discharge home visit. The therapist accompanies the patient to his own house and assesses him in his own environment. This enables her to define his need for any personal aids or adaptations to his home. The visit will often serve to give the patient confidence, to reassure the relatives, and to ensure that future plans are realistic.

Dressing is also a task in which the nurse will assist many of her patients. It is important in any ward that everyone should understand which patients will be dressed by the nurses and which will receive dressing practice from the occupational therapists.

The speech therapist

Loss of speech is not uncommon among older patients and is usually the result of a stroke. About one-third of stroke patients are affected, many of them for only a few days. But there are some who are left with severe difficulties of communication.

The speech therapist is trained to analyse the nature of the patient's speech problem and to help him overcome it.

Speech difficulties are of several kinds (though they may often occur in the same patient), difficulties of language, difficulties in word construction, weakness of the voice and difficulties in articulation.

Dysarthria

A patient with a difficulty of articulation knows the words he wishes to speak but cannot utter them clearly. This is called dysarthria. Stroke, Parkinsonism and motor neurone disease are the conditions commonly causing dysarthria in the older patient. Another common cause, at times overlooked, is loose dentures. A tin of denture fixative can improve a patient's articulation remarkably until he can see a dentist.

Verbal apraxia

Some patients know the words they want to say but get the syllables in the wrong order. They might, for example say 'ratillerpac' when they mean caterpillar. This is called verbal dyspraxia. The muscles of articulation are intact but the words are wrongly constructed.

Dysphonia

Weakness of the voice rather than speech is known as dysphonia. This is commonly due to lesions of the larynx. Dysphonia is also a feature of Parkinson's disease in the older patient.

Dysphasia

Disorders of language are known as dysphasia. Dysphasia may include a receptive as well as an expressive element, though both usually occur together. In expressive dysphasia the patient is unable to recall the word he wishes to use or he may use the wrong word. He may say no when he means yes. Or he may be able to sing or swear when he cannot speak. In receptive dysphasia the patient cannot understand what he hears. It is as if he was being addressed in a foreign language. A patient totally deprived of speech is said to be aphasic.

Helping the patient

An important part of the speech therapist's job is to explain to other members of the team and to the patient's family the nature of his disability and the best ways to help him communicate.

For example, it is important not to underestimate his comprehension or treat him as a child, still less to speak about him as if he was not there. It is important to speak clearly, not to shout. Gestures may be helpful and short sentences are best. A question that has not been understood should be rephrased. The patient must never be hurried. He needs time to reply.

The nurse must appreciate the frustration of the patient who is deprived of speech and can no longer communicate with those around him. She should try to understand his wishes and should make a point of talking to him as much as possible, as he may be able to understand though he cannot speak.

Normally a patient with speech difficulties should not be placed in a ward or day room next to a similarly disabled person. It is better, as a rule, to seat him in an area where conversation is more likely. It is possible however for a dysphasic patient to be more alone and miserable sitting in a crowded day room than in a quiet corner by himself. Occasionally two dysphasic patients, placed together, may find comfort in each other's company.

Sometimes the patient who cannot speak may be able to communicate his wishes by writing or by pointing to a picture illustrating things he might wish to do, for example having a drink or going to the lavatory. Suitable printed cards for this purpose are available from the Chest, Heart and Stroke Association (CHA). The CHA also supplies a number of helpful leaflets to assist those who are trying to help a patient with speech difficulties.

When words do begin to return the nurse should try to build the patient's confidence by encouraging him to talk as much as possible. To speak again after a stroke is like learning a new language. Much practice is needed. The nurse, as well as the speech therapist, should be prepared to explain this to the patient's relatives. They are likely to be distressed, bewildered and anxious.

Rehabilitation in the community

Rehabilitation is not always based in hospital. It is also needed by the patient at home. In some parts of Britain less than half of all those with strokes, for example, are admitted to hospital.

Some physiotherapists have always treated people outside hospital, mostly in private practice. Now more are helping patients in their own homes under the National Health Service. The primary concern of the community physiotherapist is to help the patient and his carers improve their skills in moving from bed to chair and back, walking and managing in the toilet. Her teaching gives confidence and encouragement to the carers also.

Occupational therapists also work in the community, mainly for the Social Services Department. One of their responsibilities is to advise on suitable aids and adaptations so that the patient can be as independent as possible at home. It is an advantage if the domiciliary occupational therapist can have links with her colleague in the day hospital. Together they can plan how to bridge the gap between the hospital and the community when the patient is discharged. Occupational therapists, like physiotherapists, can stimulate activity in residential homes and day centres. They can teach some of their skills to other people and so multiply their effectiveness.

The community nurse who is likely now to have had some training in geriatric rehabilitation, will work closely with the therapists and, when they are in short supply, as often happens, may take over some of their functions.

Difficulties in rehabilitation

Rehabilitation is never easy, either for the patient or the staff. But it may be made more difficult by a number of factors, mental, physical and emotional.

Mental impairment is perhaps the chief of these. The brain damage which often accompanies physical disablement in the older patient may prevent him from grasping what is required, deprive him of the will to get better or make him unrealistic about the future. Rehabilitation under these circumstances can only proceed slowly and with limited objectives.

Pain is another important obstacle and no progress may be possible until it is relieved. A painful foot for example may totally inhibit walking. Active joint disease must be treated. Analgesic drugs, intra-articular injections and the application of heat or ice by the physiotherapist may be needed.

Obesity makes all movement more difficult. Sometimes weight reduction is an essential part of rehabilitation.

Poor general condition with muscular wasting, contractures, spasticity, pressure sores and demoralisation may make rehabilitation impossible.

Emotional factors in rehabilitation

For a person to be disabled, whether suddenly as by a stroke or gradually as by arthritis or some other progressive disease, is a personal disaster. The patient will inevitably pass through a period of distress and suffering before he achieves the acceptance which enables him to co-operate in his own rehabilitation. Moreover, the effort to overcome his disability demands courage and perseverance, qualities which not everyone possesses in equal measure. Some people are endowed with optimism, resilience and persistence, while others are pessimistic, reluctant or defeatist.

No one can be rehabilitated against his will, and it is essential for the patient to have confidence in those who are looking after him. This will come more easily if he feels that they know their job, approach him with kindness and understand his problems. With a severely disabled patient time spent talking to him and listening to his problems is never wasted. Co-operation is more easily gained if the nurse has some understanding of the psychological reactions to rehabilitation and to the illness which has made it necessary.

Anxiety is perhaps the most obvious of these. The disabled patient would scarcely be human if he did not worry about his illness and about his future. He needs understanding and encouragement. If his anxieties get the better of him he may regress into childish behaviour and perhaps become incontinent. Or he may decide, consciously or subconsciously, that life in hospital is preferable to the hazards of the world outside. He will then cling to his disability as an insurance against discharge. Such a person will not be able to co-operate in his treatment. He must be encouraged to talk about his fears, and every possible step must be taken to deal with them. In this the social worker will have a large part to play.

Blame and resentment are common reactions, especially at first. 'Why did this happen to me?', 'Why does God allow it?' These are questions which no one can answer, but it is important to reassure the patient that his illness is not a punishment for past misdeeds. The disabled patient may develop a state of chronic resentment and this may focus itself on the person nearest at hand, which at home is the family and in hospital, unfortunately, the nurse. This is distressing for all concerned but the nurse should not take it personally.

Depression is an important reaction and it is perhaps the most treatable. It may show itself in the form of apathy, negativism and a reluctance to try anything new. The patient may find it impossible to believe that he can ever get better. The future seems so hopeless that he is quite unable to co-operate in rehabilitation. Such patients need appropriate treatment.

The patient's relatives and rehabilitation

The patient's illness will raise anxieties and problems for his family as well as for himself. It is important that the relatives should feel that these are appreciated by those who are treating the patient. This is mainly the province of the social worker, but the nurse can play her part by receiving the relatives with courtesy and kindness. She should answer their enquiries as far as she is able.

The relatives of the older patient are often tempted to treat him as more of an invalid than his condition justifies. They need to be kept informed of his progress and to see for themselves what he can do. Open visiting is a great help here, since the relatives often find themselves on the ward when rehabilitative activities are going on. It is far better for the visitors to see the patient walking to the lavatory, or climbing stairs, or playing bingo, than to find him tidily tucked up in bed for a traditional visiting hour.

Self-help groups

Living with disability implies adaptation to new roles, both for the patient and for those who care for him. People in this position can help each other by sharing their experiences, spreading knowledge of the problem and, perhaps, campaigning for better facilities to help the disabled. This is the basis of the increasing numbers of self-help groups such as the Parkinson's Disease Society, the Alzheimer's Disease Society and the Stroke Club Movement. Professional staff may be involved in launching these activities, but they will only succeed if the patients and those who care for them become directly involved in running the group.

For further reading:

ASSOCIATION OF CHARTERED PHYSIOTHERAPISTS IN GERIATRIC MEDICINE. 1984. *Physiotherapy with Elderly Patients*. London: Chartered Society of Physiotherapists.

CAIRD, F. I., KENNEDY, R. D. & WILLIAMS, B. O. 1983. *Practical Rehabilitation of the Elderly*. London: Pitman.

GRIFFITH, V. E., OETLIKER, P. & OSWIN, P. 1984. *A Time to Speak*. London: Chest, Heart and Stroke Association.

HAWKER, M. 1985. *The Older Patient and the Role of the Physiotherapist*. London: Faber & Faber.

RANSOME, H. 1981. *Keeping the Elderly Moving in Old People's Homes*. London: Centre for Policy on Ageing.

10
Techniques of Rehabilitation

A patient in need of rehabilitation progresses step by step. At first he may be totally dependent and able to do little or nothing for himself. Gradually he learns to do more until he achieves personal independence. The full goal of complete self-care cannot be reached by every patient, but the objective is always the fullest measure of independence possible for him and every gain, however slight, is another victory over disability.

Stages in rehabilitation

The aim of independence influences the patient's management even when he is still confined to bed. It is for this reason that so much importance is attached to the prevention of deformities and pressure sores. When the patient is in bed he should be given every opportunity to help himself. A grab handle or polly perch, suspended above the bed, may help him to move. His locker should be on his best side unless, in the case of a hemiplegic patient, a deliberate effort is being made to increase his awareness of the weak side.

The next step is to get the patient dressed and into a chair as soon as possible. This helps his morale, improves his breathing, encourages mobility and benefits his sense of balance. The only patient who should not be up for part of the day is one who is too ill to sit safely and risks falling out of the chair.

Transferring

To move from bed to chair or from chair to commode and back is called transferring. The ability to make safe transfers is fundamental to the rehabilitation of the older patient. Getting in and out of bed is further considered on pp. 141−4. Some authorities claim that a turntable is useful in helping a patient to swivel round when transferring. Others find it is one more thing to trip over and prefer not to use one.

Standing

To transfer from bed to chair the patient, unless lifted bodily, must take some weight on his legs and it may be obvious that he can stand the first time he gets out of bed. If so, all he will need is support and encouragement and perhaps a stick or walking aid to assist him. If he has been in bed for some time he may have lost his sense of balance. His trunk muscles may have become weak also.

He can be helped by the exercises of rolling and bridging. Lying on the bed, taking weight on his shoulders and on his feet, he lifts his buttocks off the mattress, a movement which will come in useful if he needs to dress in bed.

He may need to learn how to sit upright on the edge of the bed, placing his feet on the floor to improve his balance before he attempts to stand. When he has mastered this the physiotherapist may encourage his balancing reflexes by pushing him gently in various directions, saying, 'Don't let me push you over.'

Some patients need to learn how to pull themselves up from a chair, using wall bars (Fig. 5). Wall bar exercises have replaced bed end exercises which were previously advocated.

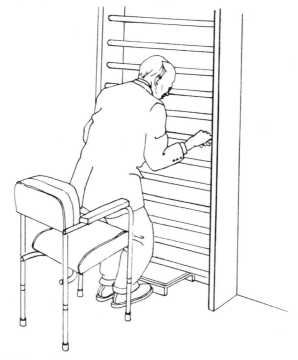

Fig. 5 At the wall bars

Getting in and out of a chair

To get into a chair is easy. As soon as the patient can feel the chair seat with the backs of his legs he puts his hands on the arms of the chair and sits down.

Getting out of a chair needs more training. The patient should support his weight on the arms of the chair until he is properly balanced on his feet. He gets up by tucking his feet backwards under the chair, throwing his weight forward and pushing himself up. Sometimes the patient clutches at a walking frame at this stage but it can give him no support. He must learn to rely only on the arms of the chair until he is on his feet. Once erect, he can grasp his walking aid first with one hand and then with the other until he is sure of his balance. Then he can move off (Fig. 6).

The nurse helping a patient to get into or out of a chair can place one foot behind the chair leg to ensure that it does not slip backwards.

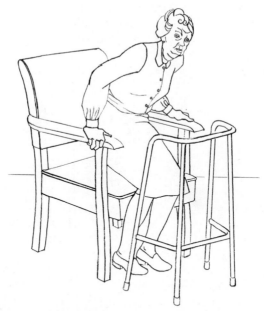

Fig. 6 Getting up from the chair

Walking

Most patients can walk a few steps as soon as they can stand. But there are some who need special help.

Walking in parallel bars

Some people may do best if they take their first steps between parallel bars (Fig. 7). Parallel bars provide firm support while the patient regains his sense of balance. If a mirror is placed at the end of the bars he can see himself walking and correct his posture as he goes.

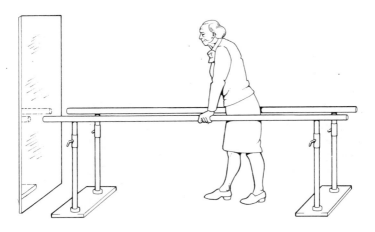

Fig. 7 Walking in parallel bars

Walking with a frame

Parallel bars are for the very disabled. Most patients can begin walking with a frame (Fig. 8a).

Frames with two front wheels like the mobilator or the Rollator give confidence in the early stages because the patient can lean on them continuously. There is no moment when he has to lift the frame from the floor. The mobilator is more generally useful because it is more compact. The Rollator provides better insurance against falling backwards but it takes up more room.

Reciprocal walking aids also provide extra stability. The frame is hinged and each side moves forward in turn. Some patients seem instinctively to prefer this method of movement.

People with weak and deformed upper limbs, usually as a result of rheumatoid arthritis, cannot grip the standard mobilator. For them the frame can be fitted with a padded platform, as in the Atlas stand aid, or with gutters, whichever is the most comfortable. The patient can then take his weight on his forearms and thus spare his wrist and hand (Fig. 8b).

The standard walking frame has no wheels and must be lifted up

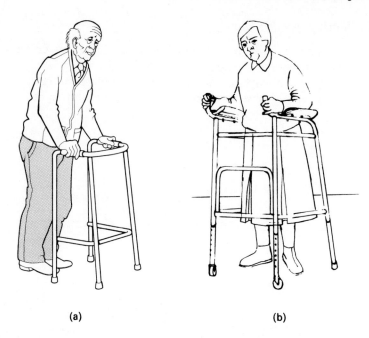

(a)   (b)

Fig. 8 (a) Walking with a frame (b) Gutter walking frame

at each step. Patients learn quickly the LIFT – PUT DOWN – LEFT FOOT – RIGHT FOOT routine and gain great confidence from it. The standard walking frame is 840 mm (33 in) high, but it is important that a variety of heights should be available and adjustable models are invaluable. The best height is that which comes up to the patient's wrist when his arm is hanging by his side.

The walking frame is suitable for any patient with a reasonable grip in both hands. Even a hemiplegic patient, if he has a little power in his upper limb, can use it to lift the walking aid and this is good training for his weak hand.

Every ward needs plenty of walking frames, not all of one kind, and if possible each patient should have his own personal frame of the correct height. Walking frames take up a good deal of room, but stackable and folding models are available which save space. Nothing however that folds is quite as reliable as a rigid model.

When the patient is learning to use the walking aid the physiotherapist or nurse should stand just behind him (Fig. 9a). She can then, if need be, hold on to the aid with him, so that he learns

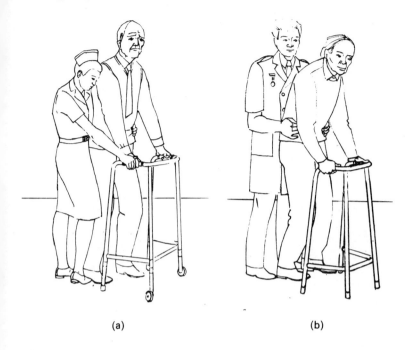

(a) (b)

Fig. 9 (a) To help a hemiplegic patient walk the nurse walks behind him, if necessary holding his hand on the mobilator
      (b) Steadying the patient from behind when he can hold a frame unaided

how to use it. Later, when he can hold the frame himself, she can steady him from behind with her hands on his hips. In this position she is well placed to support him if he stumbles or loses his balance (Fig. 9b).

Walking with a stick

A walking stick held in one hand gives most support to the opposite leg. However the patient should use the stick in whatever way he feels most comfortable. Some people are happiest with two sticks. A quadruped stick of adjustable height provides the greatest stability but the ordinary walking stick, although less stable, is lighter and more socially acceptable (Fig. 10).

The height of the stick must be adjusted to suit the patient. The handle should come to the level of the wrist when the arms hang down and the patient stands up straight. This gives a comfortable

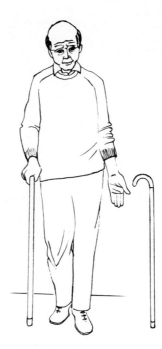

Fig. 10 The handle of a walking stick of correct length reaches the patient's wrist crease or his greater trochanter

degree of flexion at the elbow when the stick is held in the hand. The handle can be straight or curved, hard or padded, as the patient prefers. It is important that the stick should have a rubber ferrule to prevent slipping.

If possible the hemiplegic should use a walking frame rather than a stick but if he must use a stick then he should learn to use it properly. He holds it in his good hand and places it on the ground about a foot in front of him. He then leans on the stick while taking a step forward with the weak leg. Then, taking his weight on the stick and weak leg together, he brings the good leg forward. The sequence is thus STICK – WEAK LEG – GOOD LEG. As the patient gains confidence a more natural rhythm of walking can be used, the patient bringing the weak leg forward at the same moment as he advances the stick. The sequence is then STICK AND WEAK LEG – GOOD LEG – STICK AND WEAK LEG – GOOD LEG.

It is important for the nurse to understand these sequences, for the patient can be easily confused and is often tempted to advance his good leg at the same time as the walking stick. This unbalances him and he may fall. If he has a severe hemiplegia he may need support on his weak side. If not, the nurse can walk behind him and steady him with her hand on his hips.

Walking with an attendant

Some people with severe mental impairment cannot comprehend the use of a stick or walking frame. They can only walk when supported by an attendant.

Often it is best for the nurse to take the patient's arm and hold his other hand with her free hand (Fig. 11a). Another way is for the nurse to put one arm round the patient's waist, holding the hand nearest to her with her free hand. This is a good way for the patient who is very frail and needs more support (Fig. 11b).

The blind and others who need guidance rather than support often do best if they take the nurse's arm rather than vice versa. A hemiplegic patient should normally be supported from his weak side. A useful technique is for the nurse to hold the patient's weak

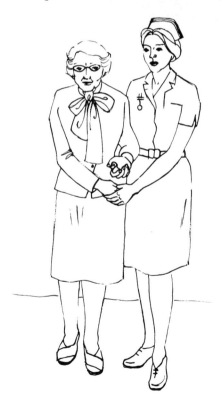

Fig. 11 (a)

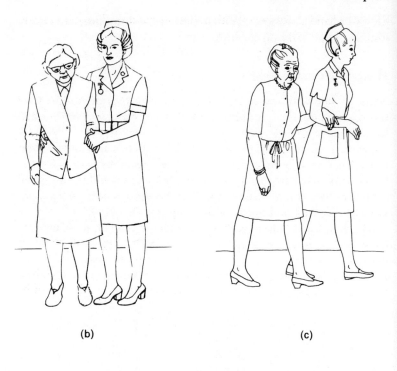

(b)

(c)

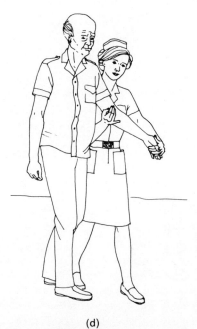

(d)

Fig. 11 Helping a frail person to walk
  (a) Cross hands grip
  (b) Waist and hand grip
  (c) Offering an arm to a blind person
  (d) Handshake grip for hemiplegic patient

hand in a hand shake grip. With her other hand she keeps his elbow straight (Fig. 11d).

Walking on stairs

Most patients can manage on the stairs once they can walk with some confidence. Patients with fixed hips and knees or poor balance have the greatest difficulties. If possible the first attempt should be made on stairs with a handrail on each side. The situation is then much the same as walking between parallel bars. A double handrail is a great advantage where the patient is hemiplegic and has only one effective hand, for he will need to use one rail for going up the stairs and the other for coming down. Where only a single handrail is available a hemiplegic patient may go up sideways, facing the banister (Fig. 12). A patient who can use both hands may prefer to use a stick in one and hold the banister with the other.

It is easier and safer to climb stairs than to descend, so a start is best made going upwards. If the patient finds the stairs at all difficult he

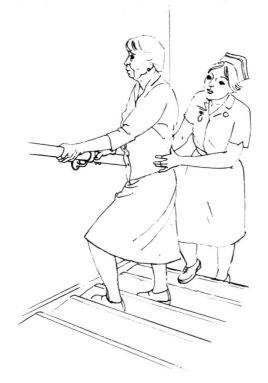

Fig. 12 Facing the banisters on the stairs

should be taught to bring both feet together on each stair. A hemiplegic patient should lead with his good leg and support himself on it while he lifts the weak leg on to the same step to join it.

When going downstairs the patient sees a big empty space below. This may alarm him. The nurse should, therefore, stand below the patient when he is coming downstairs to give him confidence and steady him if he stumbles. The hemiplegic patient when coming downstairs should lead with his weak leg, taking most of the weight on his good leg and good arm while the step is made. In this way he takes weight on the good leg while it is bent and on the weak leg only after it has been straightened.

Further points about walking

Whether he walks with the support of a nurse, or uses an aid, a stick or nothing at all, the older patient must always pay special attention to his balance. This is liable to be defective as a result of ageing alone and much more so if he has had a stroke. He should try to walk with his feet a little further apart than usual and he should take small steps. This will reduce the risk that his feet will cross over one another and trip him up.

The hemiplegic patient often finds it hard to stand up straight and because of the weakness of his trunk muscles tends to droop towards the weak side. To correct this he must learn to throw his weight towards the strong side. Sometimes it helps him to do this if the stick which he carries in his strong hand is shortened. A patient who is learning to walk should not be content to walk forwards only. As he becomes proficient he should practise walking backwards and sideways and on uneven ground as well as on the smooth floor of the ward. When he turns he should do so gradually, taking small steps. A sudden change of direction may unbalance him.

Some patients, particularly those who have not received appropriate physiotherapy from the beginning and whose leg has become spastic, develop an inversion deformity. The foot on the hemiplegic side turns inwards. The patient then walks on the outer side of the foot. As there is often foot drop as well it is very difficult for him to pick up his foot properly.

This situation used to be corrected by a caliper and T-strap which were cumbersome and unsightly. Nowadays the need for any support can usually be prevented by physiotherapy in the early stages of the stroke. The few patients whose deformity cannot be corrected in this way may be helped by a light plastic back splint which is reasonably comfortable and unobtrusive.

The wheelchair

The older patient may need a wheelchair. More than 50,000 are issued each year by the DHSS, mostly for people with arthritis, strokes and neurological disorders. A few patients, for example those with paraplegia, are completely confined to a wheelchair but most disabled elderly people can walk a few steps and use their wheelchair to extend their mobility.

There are many varieties of chair to meet varying needs in the patient and his environment. These are best considered at a Wheelchair Assessment Clinic attended by the occupational therapist, physiotherapist and technical officer from the Artificial Limb and Appliance Centre (ALAC).

The chair should be no wider than is necessary. A narrow chair goes through more doors. Some lifts and public lavatories have doors only 600 mm (24 in) wide. The seat should be the same height as any other furniture to which the patient may transfer, for example the bed, the lavatory or the commode. Detachable arm rests enable the user to slide out sideways if desired. Backrests can be of variable height and slope. Footrests must fold away and be of appropriate height. Many accessories are available including capstan hand rims, extended headrests, detachable trays, a curved mounting fitment and one arm control. There are long wheel base models for double amputees, more of whose weight is taken by the back of the chair because they lack the counter poise normally afforded by the legs. There are a variety of seats and cushions but many people prefer sheepskin.

Most chairs have the propelling wheels at the back and this is more convenient for kerbs and steps. With front wheel drive, propulsion is easier for those with stiff arms but steering is more difficult and kerbs impossible.

The most important thing for the nurse to remember about the wheelchair is that the brake should be on and the footpiece folded out of the way before the patient attempts to get in or out.

For those with weak arms (and the capacity to learn how to drive) there are a number of electric wheelchairs on the market including the Batricar which can be driven out of doors. In practice only a few elderly people learn to control any wheelchair, and fewer still an electric one. Many more depend on others to help them. For these a simple folding chair with four small wheels which goes in a car boot may be the cheapest and the most useful. Where the spouse is frail and the environment hilly an attendant controlled electric chair can be a boon, provided parking space with access to battery charging facilities is available at home (Fig. 13).

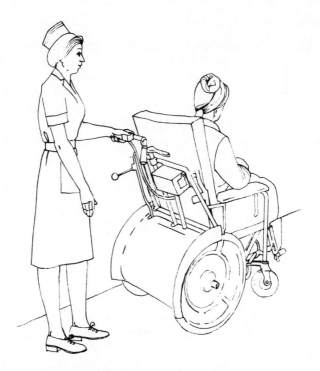

Fig. 13 Attendant controlled Model 28B wheelchair

The upper limb

In the older patient by far the commonest cause of severe disability in the upper limb is hemiplegia. After any bad stroke the arm is likely to be more affected than the leg and takes longer to recover. In the worst cases, particularly when early treatment has been lacking, the arm may become spastic, permanently paralysed and contracted. This can however usually be prevented by good physiotherapy in the early stages. The enemy, identified by Mrs Bertha Bobath, is spasticity. This can be prevented by correct positioning of the limbs from the start. When the patient is in bed lying on his weak side the arm must be extended without a pillow (Fig. 14a). When he lies on his sound side with the paralysed arm uppermost, it should be abducted and held forward on a pillow (Fig. 14b).

In a chair the patient should sit with his arm abducted, extended and pushed forward. This should become a habit whenever he is out of bed.

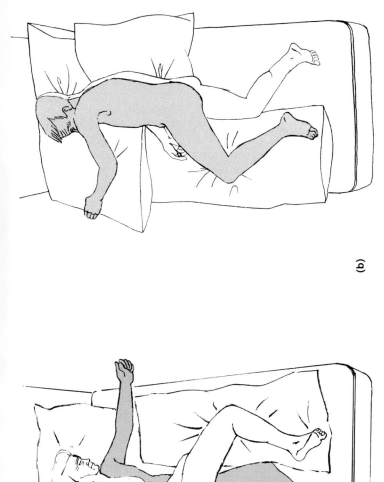

(a)

(b)

Fig. 14 Positioning the hemiplegic patient (a) Lying on the weak side (b) Lying on the sound side

The physiotherapist and the occupational therapist will give him additional exercises to overcome spasticity. These may include the application of an inflatable splint, though not all therapists believe in this.

The shoulder

After hemiplegia there is considerable risk that the patient will develop a painful frozen shoulder, but this can be prevented if the joint is never allowed to stiffen and correct positioning is maintained from the first.

In the earliest days after the stroke passive movements should be practised repeatedly. The patient can be taught to lift the weak arm with his good one, interlocking the fingers (Fig. 15). He is not likely to perform this exercise unless reminded to do so. The nurse should

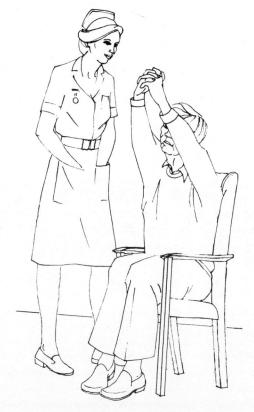

Fig. 15 Nurse encouraging the patient to do shoulder exercises

never lose an opportunity to assist him. Whenever she comes to his bed or chair she should remind him to perform this exercise, assisting him if necessary. This exercise also provides an opportunity for visitors to help. They may be glad of a chance to assist in the patient's treatment. Dressing also provides an excellent form of exercise, as it puts the shoulder through a wide range of movements.

The hand

The hand in a hemiplegic patient is the last part of the upper limb to recover and in the worst cases useful function may never be regained. In the early stages the hand will benefit if the patient tries to hold on to a walking frame, even if the nurse or physiotherapist has to hold it on for him. The contact of the hand with the frame, whenever he tries to walk, provides sensory stimulation which encourages movement and helps the patient to think two-handed. At rest the fingers should be held extended and the arm abducted to prevent spasticity. The Bexhill Arm Rest, designed by Marjorie Webster and Frances Degenhardt, is a wide detachable support which fits any chair designed to take a tray. It allows the arm to be supported in abduction and usually keeps the fingers straight (Fig. 16). If this does not prevent spasticity the fingers can be held extended by inserting them into suitably placed holes in a block of plastic foam (Fig. 16 inset).

The occupational therapist can devise activities to strengthen the hand and improve the function of the upper limb. In the early stages the aim is to help the patient to think two-handed and not to neglect the hemiplegic limb. This can be achieved by the use of a sandpapering block, saw or printing machine (Fig. 17). Later, activities can be directed to improving the control and precision of upper limb movements. Remedial games are important here, for example peg board draughts, king size dominoes and, later, solitaire, cards or jigsaw puzzles (Fig. 18).

Dressing and personal toilet are of course an important part of rehabilitation (see p. 116).

Activities of living (AL)

Thus step by step the occupational therapist re-educates the patient in the activities of living. By repeated functional assessment she studies his difficulties and tries to find ways to overcome them. This may involve the use of aids and adaptations.

In many activities one hand holds the work steady while the other

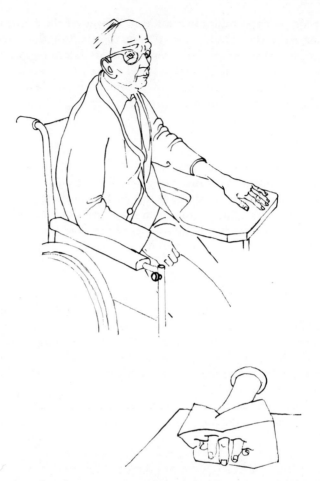

Fig. 16 Hemiplegic patient in chair with arm abducted on a Bexhill arm rest (inset) Sponge cut to keep fingers extended

performs skilled movements, for example buttering bread or peeling vegetables. Many tools are available to perform the function of holding. For example in the kitchen mixing bowls and plates can be held steady on a mat of Dycem. A can opener can be fixed to the wall. A teapot can be held in a teapot tipper. Food can be carried on a trolley rather than a tray (Fig. 19a and b). These items, once the preserve of occupational therapy departments, are increasingly available to the general public in multiple stores.

In addition there is now a wealth of electric machinery from carving knives to food processors which can be as helpful to the disabled as to the able bodied.

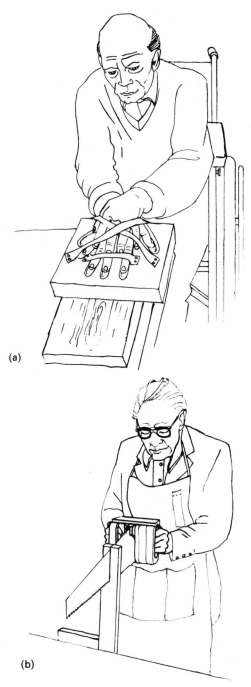

(a)

(b)

Fig. 17

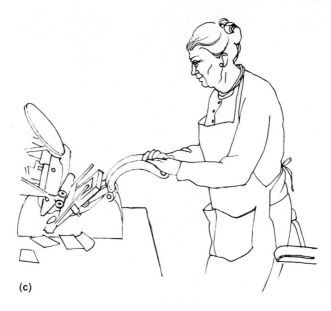

(c)

Fig. 17 Training the limb in two-handed activities
(a) Two-handed sanding block
(b) Double handled saw
(c) Two-handed printing press

Special problems in stroke patients

Some patients with strokes, even when there is no severe paralysis, fail to make progress in rehabilitation. The reason often lies in impairment of sensation, perception or comprehension, resulting from extensive damage to the brain.

The stroke may have caused dyspraxia, the inability to perform purposeful movements. Or it may have deprived the patient of postural sensation so that he loses his balance and is liable to fall. This saps his confidence and he may lose heart. Things are even more difficult if he has a hemianaesthesia with loss of all sensation in the affected limb. Or he may have a disorder of perception, hemi-agnosia. He ignores one-half of the world around him and often one-half of his own body. He may deny that a limb is paralysed or even that it belongs to him at all. He may fail to comprehend what is said to him because of sensory dysphasia. He may become withdrawn and apathetic. Much time and skill is needed to elucidate the exact nature of the patient's handicap. It is important to recognise that it is due to changes in the brain caused by the stroke.

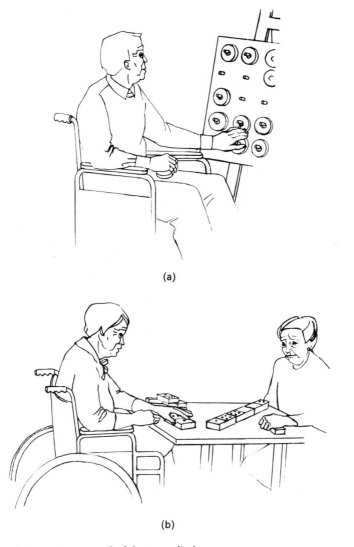

(a)

(b)

Fig. 18 Improving control of the upper limb
    (a) Peg board draughts
    (b) King size dominoes

No one must blame the patient for not trying to get better. Strokes may of course occur in patients who already have global brain damage due to dementia, but stroke itself is a rare cause of global dementia.

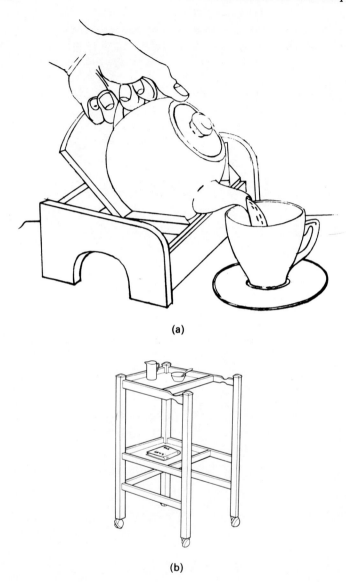

(a)

(b)

Fig. 19 Compensating for weakness in the upper limb
    (a) Teapot tipper
    (b) St. Helen's trolley

How long to treat?

A difficult problem, particularly in stroke patients, is how long to
continue physiotherapy. The evidence is that 90 per cent of

stroke patients have made their maximum recovery in three months, but this still leaves 10 per cent who will show improvement later. It is better to use the limited physiotherapy resources to treat stroke patients intensively in the early stages of their illness. If the patient is no longer improving after three months' treatment, physiotherapy should normally be withdrawn. If the situation changes later, a further course of treatment may be indicated.

For further reading:

GRASTY, P. 1985. *Home Care for the Stroke Patient*. London: Chest, Heart and Stroke Association.

HAWKER, M. 1978. *Return to Mobility*. Chest, Heart and Stroke Association.

JAY, P. E. 1980. *Help Yourselves – A Handbook for Hemiplegics and Their Families*. Sevenoaks: Butterworths.

JOHNSTONE, M. 1976. *The Stroke Patient*. Edinburgh: Churchill Livingstone.

LUBBOCK, G. (Ed). 1983. *Stroke Care – An Interdisciplinary Approach*. London: Faber and Faber.

MYCO, F. 1983. *Nursing Care of the Hemiplegic Stroke Patient*. London: Harper and Row.

II
Principles – Records – Prescriptions

The nurse, in common with all the other staff of the Department of Medicine for the Elderly, aims to help the patient regain his health, his self-respect and his place in the community. Even if he has to accept more limited objectives it should remain her aim to enable him to enjoy the best possible quality of life. To achieve this the nurse will need new knowledge, new skills and new attitudes.

Knowledge

She needs to understand something of the process of ageing. She must know about the presentation of disease in old age and the problems of multiple disability, both physical and mental. She must have an understanding of the services available to old people in the community and know about the organisation of the Department of Geriatric Medicine with its emphasis on assessment, rehabilitation and continuing care. She will come to appreciate the value of specialised equipment and the importance of good design.

Skills

The nurse who works with the elderly needs her traditional skills and adds others when in the community and in hospital. All the techniques applied on a general medical ward are used also in a geriatric ward. In addition sick old people, like others, need the nurses' skilful help with feeding, washing, toilet and general comfort. The special problem of nursing the elderly is that while the patient is often exceptionally dependent he still requires a nurse with a sense of rehabilitation who is expert in helping him to help himself. Dressing, walking and going to the lavatory are matters of the utmost importance. They provide the means whereby the patient achieves rehabilitation. The nurse becomes adept in observing the patient's appearance and mood, in assessing his function and recording what is relevant for his progress. By her sensitive awareness of occasions when the patient is disturbed or the relatives anxious she will learn to avoid confrontation and to develop good communication.

Attitudes

Knowledge and technical skill are indispensable but they are of limited value unless accompanied by the right attitude of mind. The nurse must be able to meet old age with acceptance. Not all old people are sweet tempered and grateful. Some have always been difficult and do not become any easier when they are carrying the additional burden of illness, physical handicap or mental infirmity. All must be treated with respect. It is helpful to learn as much as possible of an elderly person's past attainments, something that he is usually ready to talk about. This gives the nurse an exceptional opportunity to restore his confidence. She will not over-protect him. Rather she will see him as a unique individual with a right to function at his full potential, to make his own decisions and to take reasonable risks. She will see his disability as something to be overcome with the aid of any appliances that may help him. She will also be sensitive to his need for privacy. She will make sure that all appliances are properly used and are as inconspicuous as possible. This is particularly important with incontinence equipment and catheters, about which many patients are embarrassed.

The older patient, like the rest of the human race, feels valued when he can contribute to society. The nurse should look for opportunities for the patients to help themselves and one another. The nurse will learn to see the older patient not only as an individual but as a member of a family. His relatives and friends should be welcomed on the ward, encouraged to take part in his care and to make suggestions for its improvement. The nurse should remember that they too have their problems and want their anxieties to be appreciated. All this is easier when there is open visiting. The nurse's attitude to her colleagues is also of vital importance. In a well run hospital she should feel supported by the administration and know that any suggestion she makes for improvement in patient care will be taken seriously.

Teamwork

Finally she will see herself as one of a multidisciplinary team to which each member makes her own expert contribution. Besides the nurse the team includes doctors, social workers, physiotherapists and occupational therapists, remedial gymnasts and housekeepers.

All these people share a common core of knowledge about the older patient but they bring also their own professional expertise and understanding. There is, therefore, a considerable area of overlap in their approach to the patient, particularly in the day room. All are trying to help the patient as an individual. The nurse should feel ready to sit down and play a game with the patient or join him in a cup of tea. Equally an occupational therapy helper, for example, will be ready to help the patient in the lavatory or with his dressing. This blurring of roles is to be encouraged. There is no room for an exclusive or possessive attitude. One of the pleasures of caring for the elderly is the experience of working in a close knit team.

Care Planning

The medical and nursing notes provide the foundation on which the patient's care is planned. The nursing problems are listed in order of priority.

Urgent problems

The nurse is the first person to see the patient when he is admitted and must decide how urgent is the need to summon the doctor. Symptoms demanding immediate action include severe dyspnoea, pain, collapse, haemorrhage and loss of consciousness. In these situations action must be taken at once and notes may have to be made later.

In many old people, especially the most ill and most immobile, the care plan must take account of the high risk of pressure sores and appropriate preventive measures instituted. Patients with strokes will require positioning in ways which reduce spasticity. Most patients are apprehensive and will be reassured if the nurse explains what she is doing and what is likely to happen next.

Symptom relief

What the nurse and doctor perceive as the most important problems are not always those that most concern the patient. For example, a person with advanced cancer may be much troubled by an itching skin or a sore mouth or constipation or worried about her home. Sometimes the patient is hesitant to mention these things and the relatives should be encouraged to draw the attention of the staff towards them. The staff need to understand as much as possible of the patient's personality, tastes and habits. To some people interference with the routines of living can be a source of much distress.

Rehabilitation

The care plans for the patient in acute illness must take into account his needs as a whole person and particularly his need for mobility. The wrong sort of care can rob a patient of his independence. The right care plan will ensure that every effort is made to preserve the patient's independence, mobility and self-respect.

For example, the patient should be dressed in his own clothes from an early stage in his illness. At first he may need much help but gradually he should do more for himself. Another vital goal for the patient is to walk to the lavatory and to attend to his own toilet needs. The surgeon, Mr M. B. Devas, has a saying well worth pondering, 'The first step in rehabilitation is the first step.'

Evaluation

Each stage in the patient's rehabilitation must be identified and recorded. This is the third phase of the nursing process, evaluation. It leads to reassessment and revision of the care plan and highlights the importance of the nursing records.

Nursing records

The medical and nursing notes provide information which is available to all members of the team. The nursing process promotes a consistent approach to the patient by everyone involved. This is especially important during the period when assistance is being withdrawn from the patient in order to encourage him to do more for himself.

These records go with the patient wherever he moves within the department or when he is transferred to the care of another specialist.

Verbal communication

Good written records are only one aspect of communication with the ward team. The spoken word is equally important especially in wards where many patients are too ill or too confused to make their wishes clear. The change over is a key moment, when the nurse going off-duty hands over to the colleague who is relieving her. As well as receiving the report in the office the oncoming nurse-in-charge should be introduced personally to anyone newly admitted. This makes the patient feel more secure.

Temperature charts

In wards for the elderly all temperatures should be taken with wide range thermometers reading from 25 °C to 40 °C. Mouth readings are best if the patient can co-operate but the temperature should be confirmed rectally if the mouth reading is below 35 °C. Few patients need to have their temperature recorded more than once a day. The late afternoon is the most useful time because this is when the temperature is highest. Very ill patients should have the temperature recorded four-hourly for the first twenty-four hours after admission. Those with hypothermia will need hourly readings until the temperature returns to normal. In such patients the temperature should be taken rectally, and a special chart is needed.

Temperature taking can safely be discontinued when the patient is no longer acutely ill. In rehabilitation and continuing care wards temperatures are only taken if the patient looks unwell.

The pulse too should be recorded whenever the temperature is taken. The significance of the pulse rate in the elderly is the same as in younger patients.

The respiration rate of the older patient is particularly informative and special efforts should be made to record this accurately. The best way to do this is for the nurse to adjust her own breathing to that of the patient, while she counts. An increased rate is often the first sign of pneumonia.

Fluid charts

It is difficult and time consuming to maintain accurate fluid charts in a ward for the elderly but inaccurate fluid records are useless. Unnecessary fluid charting, therefore, should be avoided. The recording of fluid intake is essential only when the patient is on an intravenous or subcutaneous drip, and it must be noted with the utmost care.

If the patient is incontinent his urinary output can only be recorded if he is catheterised. If he is receiving diuretics his response to treatment is monitored better by weighing him than attempting to measure his urine.

Weighing

Records of the patient's weight are important as a guide to progress. Every ward for the elderly, including continuing care units, should have a chair-type weighing machine. Long-stay patients should be weighed monthly, others every week or fortnight. The weight should be recorded in the medical or nursing case notes. It should not be written on the temperature chart since this is likely to be discontinued before the patient leaves hospital. Some skill is required to weigh an elderly patient accurately. The patient should sit upright in the middle of the chair. If he leans too far backwards or slumps forward large variations in his weight may be recorded. The correct weight is shown when the bar floats horizontally between the stops.

Blood pressure records

Blood pressure records, sometimes at frequent intervals, may be needed when the patient is shocked or collapsed. On the other hand it is easy for these records, once started, to run on much longer than is necessary. The nurse should always be ready to ask how long the doctor requires them to be continued.

The older patient with hypertension is seldom treated with powerful hypotensive drugs, so much blood pressure recording which is common in general medical wards is avoided in wards for the elderly. On the other hand some elderly people, especially if under treatment with tranquillisers or antidepressant drugs, may suffer from postural hypotension. In these patients it may be necessary to record the blood pressure lying, standing and sitting.

Bowel records

Because of the older patient's tendency to constipation and the risk of faecal impaction it is necessary to keep a record of his bowel action in the nursing notes. For patients with diarrhoea a stool chart is indispensable. This is kept at the end of the patient's bed. Every stool passed is recorded immediately by the nurse who attends the patient. The chart should be ruled off at the end of each day.

Other charts

Special charts should be used for patients whose next dose of drugs depends on information from the laboratory. Anticoagulants are the main example here but the same problem arises with drugs which affect the blood count, mainly those used in the chemo-therapy of malignant disease.

Prescriptions

Every hospital has its own ideas about prescription charts and it is important to the nurse that they should be satisfactory. Medicine rounds normally take place at fixed times, usually 8 a.m., 12 noon, 4 p.m. and 10 p.m. The doctor must be persuaded to write his prescription in block capitals, preferably using the drug's generic name, and indicating the dose, the route of administration, the times it has to be given and for how long. Prescription sheets should be of a type in which every dose can be recorded as it is given. It is part of the nurse's job to persuade the doctors, particularly the junior doctors who change so often, to collaborate in following the department's prescribing policy. In long-stay units it is particularly important for prescriptions to be reviewed regularly. It is only too easy for a patient to receive drugs week after week and month after month when they have ceased to be necessary.

Medicine rounds take a long time in a ward for the elderly. With increasingly rapid turnover the problems of ensuring that the right drug is given to the right patient become ever more difficult. It is vital to identify each patient by checking his name before the drugs are given. To avoid mistakes the round should be done by two people. The nurses should not only give out the tablets but check that the patient takes them. On occasion a patient may refuse his medication. If so, the nurse should record the fact. Medicine should not be added to food or drink as this may make the patient refuse all nourishment. A suspicious person may fear that he is being poisoned.

All drugs have side effects and the nurses are often the first person to suspect them. They include confusion, giddiness, skin rashes, drowsiness, nausea and vomiting. The nurse's observations are of particular value in deciding the best dose of tranquilliser for the restless patient or of an analgesic for someone in pain.

Drugs in the Day Hospital

The older patient, when he attends the Day Hospital, may be receiving drugs from both his general practitioner and from the hospital. It is important that each is aware of the drugs prescribed by the other. The patient should carry a communication card on which each doctor writes details of any treatment he has ordered.

What the patient is actually taking is another matter. He should be asked to bring all his medicines with him to the Day Hospital, so that the nurse can check them with him. This will help him to understand how to take the right medicines in the right dose at the right time.

For further reading:

MACDONALD, E. T. & MACDONALD, J. B. 1982. *Drug Treatment in the Elderly*. Chichester: John Wiley.

MACFARLANE, J. & CASTLEDINE, G. 1982. *A Guide to the Practice of Nursing Using the Nursing Process*. St. Louis: Mosby.

ROYAL COLLEGE OF PHYSICIANS. 1984. *Medication for the Elderly*. Royal College of Physicians.

12
The Patient's Day —
Dressing — Nutrition

The patient's day should be as much like a normal day at home as possible. This is easier to preach than to practise since inevitably its pattern is a compromise between the varying needs of many patients, the availability of staff at different times, the size of the day area and the number and siting of toilet facilities.

Old people should be out of bed as much as possible but this should not become a fetish. Those who look ill or overtired or who ask to go back to bed should normally do so, but some will want to get up again later. There are many for whom a rest on their beds after lunch is very acceptable. To sit too long in a chair without moving can be very tiring. Even moves from bed to chair and chair to bed break up the monotony and provide exercise.

Early morning

Many old people are used to waking early and are glad when their first cup of tea arrives about 7 a.m. Those who are not awake should be allowed to sleep later if circumstances allow. All patients need toileting when they first wake and many wet beds occur because of the difficulty of attending to patients without delay at this time.

In the day room

After breakfast the patient will be toileted and helped to dress. If at all possible he should wash in the bathroom. Once dressed and wearing proper shoes he should go to the day room, where a planned programme of activities will be in operation. Many patients require specific physiotherapy and occupational therapy. Most should join in exercises to music designed to improve mobility, and in games, craftwork and diversional activities to stimulate the mind. After lunch most people enjoy a siesta. The ideal is a balanced programme of activity and rest tailored to the needs and wishes of each individual. In practice there must be a good deal of give and take. For the very frail a short day of about six hours with a fair amount of activity is better than a longer inactive day.

Background music, although popular with the nurses, is seldom acceptable to the older patient and makes it harder for the deaf. Music for specific purposes such as group exercises, community singing or religious services is a different matter and is much enjoyed. Television should be switched on for particular programmes only. It is especially enjoyed in the evenings by those who do not like to go to bed too early. Every effort should be made to meet their wishes.

All these activities are equally appropriate to the geriatric day hospital. In some units the inpatients day room and the outpatients day hospital are one and the same. In such an environment the nurse has a special opportunity to work with other members of the team. In so doing she will have new opportunities to observe her patient's response and to understand him.

Visiting

An important part of the patient's day is to see his visitors. They provide both stimulation and support as well as keeping him in touch with his home. Many relatives will have cared for the patient at home and may want to feel part of the caring team in hospital. Their confidence will be increased if they can spend time on the ward and see as much as possible of what goes on. The nurse should be ready to offer them opportunities to participate in the patient's care, should they wish to do so.

Back to bed

The patient should as far as possible choose his own bedtime, though this is not easy when there are few nurses on the evening shift. It may be possible for him to undress and wash early in the evening and to have supper in his dressing gown, perhaps watching television afterwards. When he goes to bed he may need a nightcap to help him settle, a milky drink or alcohol, which has a sedative effect. Sleeping tablets are better avoided. If they must be used they should be given early in the evening or the patient will be drowsy next morning and sleep badly the following night.

At night

An important part of the night nurse's duty is to continue the two-hourly turning of patients who are judged to be at risk for pressure sores. This is hard to achieve unless the establishment allows at least two nurses to be on duty in each ward at the same time.

Good night care makes an important contribution to the patient's rehabilitation and a particularly important task of the night nurse is toileting. The way in which this is done can improve a patient's mobility, continence and self-respect. The nursing history should show how often the patient normally goes to toilet in the night and as far as possible this pattern should be maintained. The patient's bed should be in a low position so that he can easily get in and out. He should be reminded how to summon help and the call bell must be within reach. Some patients will be kept dry only if they are woken by the nurse several times during the night. A few, usually those with severe brain damage, may require a catheter or diapers. But this is a treatment of last resort (see Ch. 18).

The confused, noisy or restless old person is the night nurse's most difficult problem. There are many reasons for acute confusion (see p. 228) but it is always worth checking that the patient does not have a wet bed, a full bladder, an overloaded rectum or pain for some other reason. The frightened patient often responds to a reassuring word, accompanied perhaps by a cup of tea. If he wants to be up he should be allowed to do so and safety sides should not be used to restrain him. If a confrontation can be avoided the patient will usually be glad to go back to bed quite quickly and peace will be restored to the ward. Where simple measures fail the doctor must be consulted. The best solution may be to move the patient to a single room if there is one.

Night wear

Unless he is very incontinent the patient should wear his own night clothes. If this is not possible the hospital will supply nightgowns or pyjamas. Good night wear should be easy to put on with deep armholes and loose sleeves. It is an affront to the patient's dignity to nurse a man in a pyjama jacket only, but night shirts, now increasingly fashionable, are sometimes welcome. The open back nightgowns, previously advocated for patients with a tendency to incontinence, are now mainly used for the unconscious or acutely ill patient who must be nursed entirely in bed.

Dressing

Dressing is an important event in the patient's day and should form part of the treatment of all but the most ill old people. Not only is it a good form of physiotherapy, exercising every joint in the body, but it has an excellent psychological effect. There is a strong association between getting dressed and getting better. This helps not only the patient but his relatives and the hospital staff. Everyone feels it immediately.

Clothing expresses our personality and to enable her patient to wear his own clothes is one of the most powerful ways in which a nurse can preserve his individuality. To be dressed in clothes of our own choice is vital to self-esteem. On the other hand to wear clothes from a communal stock is humiliating and degrading. It takes effort for the nurse to keep a patient dressed in his own clothes and will involve regular contact with his visitors. But well-dressed patients and their relatives are likely to be more content and this will contribute to job satisfaction among the staff.

Clothes

The patient's clothes should never be removed from the ward. To have them at hand gives a feeling of security, and their removal causes needless concern. The conventional bedside locker is not designed for storing clothes and suitable furniture for this purpose should be provided for every patient (see p. 157).

Sometimes there is difficulty in getting suitable shoes and these may need to be bought. A light lace up or strap shoe is usually best. Where the feet are swollen or deformed felt boots are invaluable. They are available in a variety of colours with laces or velcro fastenings. The heel can be raised if necessary.

Helping the patient to dress

As far as possible the patient should attend to his own dressing, but some help may be needed. Patients normally dress as soon as they get up. The nurse should make sure that all their clothes are put out for them in the proper order. She will probably need to help them with their underwear, trousers, stockings and shoes. It may help to rest the foot on a stool.

Difficulties in dressing

The occupational therapist is the expert in the assessment of dressing difficulties. It is part of her job to suggest solutions. The nurse will learn from her at ward case conferences and from studying the nursing or medical notes.

Dressing may become difficult for many reasons. A weak limb or a stiff joint is a common cause. Patients with a bad arm should put it into the sleeve first. In undressing the good arm is removed from the sleeve first. People with stiff hips and knees have difficulty with shoes and stockings. Long-handled shoehorns and stocking aids may help them (Fig. 20 a and b). A dressing stick, straight or curved with a padded end, can be used to hold a garment over the head in dressing or to push one off a weak shoulder in undressing (Fig. 20 c). It has a hook on the unpadded end useful for zip fasteners and for picking things off the floor. The patient with poor eyesight can be helped if part of a garment which is to be put on first is identified by a marker. For example a large white patch can be put in the armhole of a dress or jacket. The patient with brain damage, Parkinsonism or vertebrobasilar insufficiency may be very unsteady on his feet. His problem is usually solved if he will dress sitting down. More extensive brain damage can cause apraxia. The patient loses all idea of dressing even though his limbs may not be paralysed. Other patients may simply have poor memory. They get into a muddle because they forget what to do next. They need a lot of supervision with repeated reminders at every stage of dressing. All this demands great patience of the nurse. The patient may find dressing difficult because of breathlessness or exhaustion due to failure of the heart

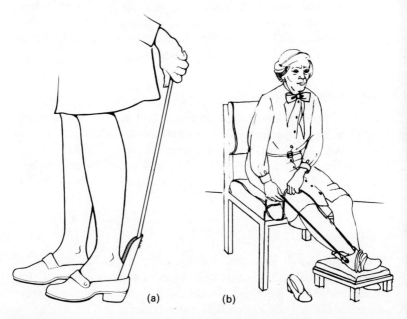

(a)   (b)

Fig. 20 a, b

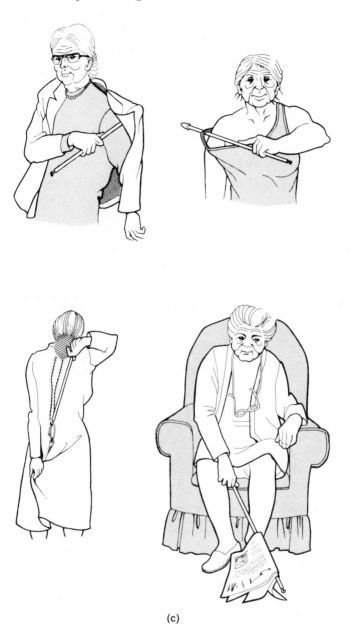

(c)

Fig. 20 Dressing aids
    (a) Long-handled shoe horn
    (b) Stocking aid
    (c) Dressing stick used to get a coat off the shoulder, manipulate a
        shoulder strap, pull a zip fastener, pick a paper off the floor

and lungs. Or he may simply give up the struggle from depression and despair. Medical treatment and encouragement by the nurse may overcome this. Several of these difficulties may affect patients who have had a stroke and all the problems listed above may be present in one patient.

Suitable clothes

The older patient should wear the clothes he likes, but the more disabled he is the more likely it becomes that his clothing will be determined by his handicap. People who are unsteady on their feet feel insecure while putting garments over their head, so cardigans are better than pullovers. Front fastening dresses and coat-type shirts are also advisable. Wrap-round skirts are liked by many elderly women. If more men were allowed by fashion to wear kilts like Scotsmen, life would be easier for them in old age. Trousers with deepened fly openings help men to use a bottle sitting down. Separates are useful for people confined to wheelchairs. A jacket split down the centre back seam is easier to put on when the user is seated. Clothes for the disabled should have deep armholes and wide sleeves. Where narrower sleeves are preferred they should be lined with low friction material such as silk or nylon. Velcro can be used for fastening shirts, trousers, dresses, bras, ties and belts, but it is not suitable for use with woollen garments. Buttons, if used at all, should be large and easy to grasp. The right accessories are also useful. They may include clip-on aprons and braces, made-up ties and expanding cuff links. Special clothing for the incontinent such as split-back skirts has become less important with recent improvements in protective underclothing (see p. 206).

Clothing co-ordinator

Most patients have relatives who will be able to purchase new clothes and arrange for laundering as they would if the old person was being cared for at home. However, especially in long-stay units, there will always be a few patients whose families cannot provide this service. The responsibility will then fall on the hospital. The patient's pension will provide the finance for clothes but he will need help to purchase suitable garments. He can be taken out to the shops or a firm can bring a selection to the hospital. Some firms, for example, Bowens Bros., specialise in this service.

All clothing should be marked. Laundering can be done in the hospital if the hospital laundry is equipped to deal with personal clothing. Alternatively a ward unit can be equipped with its own washing machine and drying cabinet. In many hospitals the ward launderette can be run by the housekeeping team but some large long-stay hospitals have found it valuable to appoint a clothing co-ordinator to run the service.

Nutrition

Eating remains a pleasure that the older patient can enjoy to the end of his days. His food, therefore, makes an important contribution to his quality of life and must be of concern to the nurse. People over 75 at home require about 2 000 Kcal (8.3 MJ). In hospital, although food is plentiful, appetites are often poor and many patients take only about 1 500 Kcal (6.25 MJ) a day.

Vitamins

Old people who are housebound because of physical illness and disability, mental disorder or social isolation eat less than their more active contemporaries and are more likely to suffer from malnutrition. The commonest deficiency is lack of Vitamin D. A poor dietary intake is only one factor in this. Malabsorption may contribute but lack of exposure to sunlight is probably the main factor. Institutional cooking destroys a good deal of Vitamin C but serious deficiency is rare. Lack of Vitamin B is also uncommon. Some old people are deficient in potassium and folic acid which are present mainly in fruit, cereals and green vegetables. Potassium deficiency is more likely when the patient is taking diuretics.

Fibre

Fibre is now recognised as an essential part of a healthy diet but many old people are not accustomed to eating enough of the foods which contain it. The main sources of fibre are wholemeal bread, bran based biscuits and cereals, root vegetables and fruit. Many of the most popular foods, white bread, sugar, biscuits, cakes and sweets consist mainly of carbohydrate and are fattening.

Obesity

It is not surprising, therefore, that the commonest form of nutritional disorder in the elderly, as in the rest of the population, is obesity. This contributes to many illnesses.

Presentation of food

Food has not only to contain the right nutrients and to be well prepared. It must arrive in the ward hot and be served attractively. It must also be presented in ways which are acceptable to the patient. Many old people have no difficulty in using a knife and fork and can eat as they always have done. For the very frail, however, things are different. For example, boiled eggs and oranges are excellent foods but a boiled egg needs the top removed and an orange needs peeling before it can be eaten. These may be impossible tasks for a patient with shaky hands or a hemiplegia. Such foods are better served in other ways. Fruit may be chopped or set in jelly or the juice may be offered as a drink. Bacon and fish are important sources of protein but some old people may choke on the bacon rind or on a fish bone which they have failed to see. Bacon should, therefore, have the rind removed before it is served and fish must be carefully filleted. Fish fingers are particularly suitable. If a patient has only one effective hand any form of food requiring both a knife and fork will be beyond him. Food must be cut up and it is better to serve dishes that can be eaten with one implement only. Meat should either be minced so that it can be eaten with a spoon or else served in chunks which can be picked up with a fork. Sausages should be skinless and vegetables mashed or diced. Pureed foods are very acceptable to those who find it difficult to chew. Soup, served in a cup, and sandwiches are popular for supper. Most people prefer a continental breakfast.

Choice of food

Choice is a vital ingredient in anyone's quality of life. An advance in hospital catering has been the introduction of menu cards on which the patient may indicate his choice of food from two or three alternatives. Many old people will need help from the nurse to complete their cards. The nurse should see the time spent doing this as a way of reinforcing the patient's individuality, even if, by the time the food arrives, he cannot remember what he ordered. The system can operate equally well with meals plated in the kitchen or served on the ward. At present a choice of food is more often available in hospital than in residential homes.

Methods of feeding

Whenever possible the older patient should be out of bed for meals. He should wear his dentures and the nurse should observe whether they fit properly. The patient should not eat off a tray in his armchair but at a dining table with two or three others to facilitate conversation. The table should be properly laid with a cloth or place mats. Even if meals are served plated, the condiments should be provided for each table. Tea should be served from small pots, one for each table, and not from a communal urn.

If the patient is hemiplegic the food should be placed so that he can reach it with his good hand. A person with one effective hand manages better if the food is served in a soup bowl or a plate with a raised rim. An ordinary plate can be made serviceable with a bunker (Fig. 21a). The plate can be steadied on a mat of non-stick plastic. At home a meal can be carried on a trolley or served on a tray with a Dycem non-slip surface (Fig. 21b). Flexible plastic egg cups with a suction base can be obtained. The Nelson combined knife and fork and the Spork, combined spoon and fork, are invaluable for hemiplegic patients (Fig. 21c). Patients with weak hands may be helped by cutlery with expanded handles. A convenient method is to slip the handles into a length of rubazote or foam rubber tubing. This can readily be removed for washing up. Occasionally patients with stiff elbows and shoulders may find it easier to feed themselves if the spoon has an angled end or a lengthened handle (Fig. 21c). For those whose hands are shaky a teacher beaker is helpful (Fig. 21d). If necessary a flexible straw can be inserted through the lid. The Manoy mug is specially adapted for weak hands (Fig. 21e).

It is important to make sure that the patient finds these aids acceptable. He should always be given the choice before he has to use them and he should not be compelled to do so against his will.

Napkins

The older patient, with perhaps poor eyesight and an unsteady hand, may be a messy eater, particularly when he is not at a table. The temptation to give him a bib to protect his clothing is considerable and there are large plastic bibs available with a trough to catch the crumbs and spillage. Bibs, however, are likely to be felt as an affront to the patient's dignity. It is better to use a napkin tucked into the neck as is done all over the continent. The Kleenex nursing roll provides napkins of suitable size. Disposable protective serviettes are also available, but cost more.

Feeding the helpless patient

No one should be fed who is capable of feeding himself. To be fed returns the patient to babyhood and is the ultimate denial of his independence. Even so there are likely in any ward to be some patients so ill or so helpless that they require feeding. If so the nurse should sit down so that the patient feels she has plenty of time. Feeding is a job very suitable for relatives, some of whom may be glad to take a direct part in the patient's care. Their assistance should always be welcomed.

Fluid

Even more important for the older patient than his feeding is attention to his fluid balance. Old people who are ill do not always

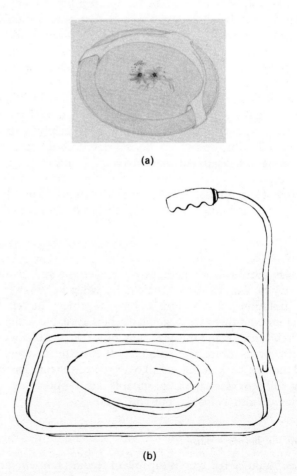

(a)

(b)

Fig. 21 a, b

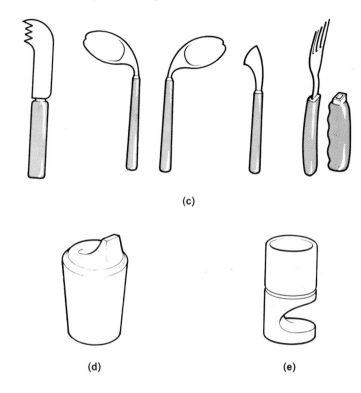

(c)

(d)   (e)

Fig. 21 Aids for eating and drinking
(a) Plate with bunker
(b) Manoy dish with one straight and one sloping side. One-handed tray with Dycem non-slip surface
(c) (left to right) Nelson knife, left- and right-handed Manoy spoons, one-handed knife, fork with expanded handle
(d) Teacher beaker
(e) Manoy mug with base designed for grip by weak hand

feel thirsty or drink as much as they should. They may very readily become dehydrated. The older patient requires about two litres of liquid in 24 hours, though this may be increased if there is fever, sweating, polyuria or dehydration. Normally about one litre of water is included in his food, leaving another litre to be provided as drink. This is amply covered if the patient will take every cup of tea or coffee normally offered to him and empty a jug containing half a litre left by his bedside. If the patient is not eating, then the full two litres must be provided. The nurse should never remove un-consumed drink from the patient's bedside without making an effort to get him to drink some of it.

Drinking difficulties

It is, however, often hard for the patient to drink all that he should. Some people, usually women, drink very little in order not to have to empty their bladder at night. Others may find the effort to drink too much for them when they are ill. Others again may have difficulty in swallowing or if confused may forget to drink. Those who are unconscious or unable to speak cannot tell the nurse that they are thirsty.

Urine output

The older patient cannot easily compensate for a small fluid intake by excreting less urine. With advancing years the kidneys lose some of their concentrating power and are unable to produce urine of a high specific gravity. The patient thus continues to lose fluid when he can least afford it. If in addition there is vomiting or diarrhoea, leading to loss of salts as well as water, it becomes doubly hard for the older patient to maintain his fluid balance.

The patient with dysphagia

Patients who have difficulty in swallowing are often better if they do not attempt to drink, but take their liquids in a semi-solid form. For example, milk, drinks and soups can be thickened. Ice cream is popular and so are ice lollies. Jellies, yoghurt and purees are all convenient. A liquidiser is useful in the ward kitchen.

Gastric drips are not suitable for patients with dysphagia. There is a great risk of regurgitation and inhalation of the gastric contents. Such patients should be given their fluid parenterally.

Parenteral fluid

As the patient will not be taking other food at least two litres of fluid (more if the patient is dehydrated) will need to be given in 24 hours either intravenously or by subcutaneous infusion. A litre of normal saline and a litre of 5 per cent dextrose each given over 12 hours will usually suffice. 4.3 per cent dextrose in one-fifth normal saline is an alternative. If there is potassium deficiency, potassium chloride will be added to the drip.

A litre of fluid given over 24 hours represents a drop rate of 12 drops per minute. If, for example, it is intended to give the patient two litres in 24 hours, changing the unit every 12 hours, this will be achieved with a drip rate of 24 drops per minute.

For further reading:

DEAN, F. 1982. *Clothing Needs of the Elderly Person.* Disabled Living Foundation.

RUSTON, R. 1982. *Dressing for Disabled People.* Disabled Living Foundation.

TURNBULL, P. 1982. *A Guide to the Introduction of a Personal Clothing Service.* Disabled Living Foundation.

WADE, B., SAWYER, L. & BELL, J. 1983. *Dependency with Dignity.* London: Bedford Square Press.

13
Moving and Lifting

An ill patient should be nursed either nearly flat or as upright as possible with his feet well supported to stop him slipping down the bed. An overhead 'grab handle' may help him to retain a good position. More useful at home perhaps is a rope ladder attached to the bed end. A semi-recumbent posture should be avoided as it increases the shearing strain on the skin of the back and predisposes to pressure sores. These considerations do not apply if the patient can move freely or if he is being nursed on a bed with a hinged section.

Lifting the patient up the bed

When lifting the patient up the bed it is important to avoid friction since this may cause abrasions of the back and heels. Good techniques of lifting are therefore important. It is easier to lift heavy weights when these are held close to the body and the nurse should always get close to the patient. Lifting should always be done by movements of the legs while the back itself is kept as straight as possible. Never to lift with a bent back is the nurse's best insurance against injury. These principles are most effectively embodied in the shoulder lift. For the shoulder lift the patient must be sitting up (Fig. 22). The two nurses stand with bent knees and slightly flexed hips facing one another across the bed at the level of the patient's pelvis. Their bodies and feet are turned a little towards the head of the bed. Each nurse passes one arm beneath the patient's thighs and grasps her partner's wrist (Fig. 22 inset). The double wrist grip is the best way for nurses to join their arms when lifting. The other arm is pressed down on to the mattress, well up towards the bed head. Each nurse then presses her shoulder into the axilla of the patient, who rests an arm on each of their backs. At an agreed word the nurses straighten their legs and thus lift the patient with their shoulders, taking most of their weight on the leg nearest the end of the bed. By transferring the weight to the other leg the nurses move the patient up the bed. The shoulder lift is unsuitable for those with disease or injury of the chest, shoulders or arms.

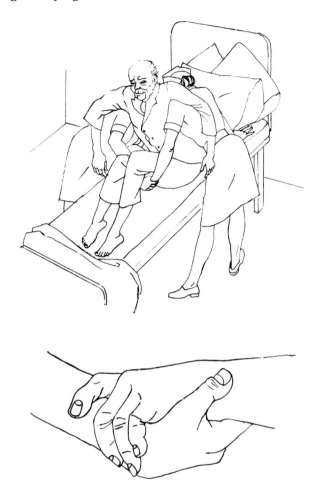

Fig. 22 Shoulder lift
(Inset) Double wrist grip

Draw-sheet lift

Where the shoulder lift cannot be used, the draw-sheet lift may be employed. The patient is helped into a sitting position on his draw-sheet. Two nurses grasp the corners of the draw-sheet and, using their legs and body weight, move the patient up the bed in short lifts.

If the patient is too heavy to be moved easily by two nurses a hoist should be used.

Mary Rose sling

The draw-sheet type of lift or the Australian lift may be made
easier by the Mary Rose sling (Jarvis Leather Goods, 116 Seaside,
Eastbourne, East Sussex). Inspired by the raising of the ship, the
Mary Rose, the sling is promoted as 'a handle on a patient'. The
sling is placed under the patient's upper thighs. It provides a
convenient hand hold for the nurses to grasp when they wish to lift
him up the bed or chair and has proved most acceptable (Fig. 23).

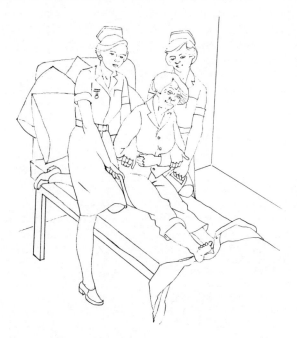

Fig. 23 Using the Mary Rose sling

Getting up

The daily nursing care of the older patient comprises not only
rest, which is needed by any sick person, but also a suitable measure
of activity. It is not merely that some activity is good for the older
patient. It is essential to his survival as a self-respecting human being.
Old people go off their legs very readily and once the ability to walk
is lost, it can be a long struggle to regain it. To keep an old person in
bed without grave reason is likely to induce a state of apathy and
mental deterioration, usually accompanied by incontinence. Bedfast

patients become feeble and their joints become stiff. They may develop contractures and they are liable to pressure sores.

Getting the patient up takes time, but nothing is more important for his welfare. To leave him in bed without very good reason is a form of neglect. In a geriatric ward it should be regarded as normal for the patient to be up and exceptional for him to be in bed. To understand this is perhaps the most important single step in learning to care for the older patient.

A modern geriatric ward, used for rehabilitation or continuing care, should be thought of primarily as a day unit with beds. It is particularly important that separate sitting and dining areas are available so that the patient can move from one to the other from time to time during the day.

Helping the patient out of bed

Before getting a patient out of bed, it is important to have the furniture in the proper position. The chair or commode should be near the bed. If the patient is hemiplegic, it is best to place it on his good side at first. As he improves, however, he should learn to approach it with his weak side also. The adjustable height bed should be in a suitably low position and the wheels should be braked. The nurse helps the patient to swing his legs over the edge of the bed until he is sitting upright with his feet on the floor (Fig. 24). Once he is seated on the edge of the bed, he should pause while he gets his balance. The nurse can help him adjust his clothing and put his shoes on at this stage. She then assists him to his feet. This can be

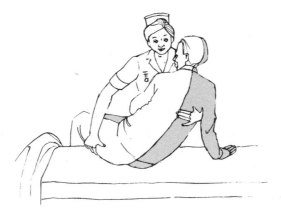

Fig. 24 Helping the hemiplegic patient out of bed

done in two ways. If the patient is reasonably mobile, she will be able to help him from the side, putting one hand across his back and the other supporting him by the hand, elbow or shoulder. By placing one foot in front of the patient's toes she can ensure that he will not slip as he stands up.

A heavy patient needing more support is better approached from the front. Facing the patient the nurse places her arms under his axillae with her hands on his shoulder blades. He puts his arms around her neck. Keeping her back straight she presses her bent knees against his and by straightening her legs brings him to his feet using her weight as a counterbalance (Fig. 25). This may be made easier by rocking the patient to and fro before the lift is made.

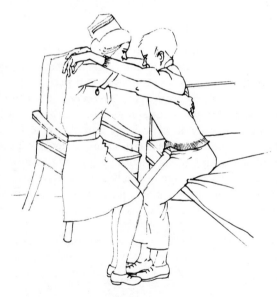

Fig. 25 Helping the patient from bed to chair

Once he is on his feet she helps the patient to turn until he can feel the chair seat at the back of his legs. As soon as possible he should learn to reach with his hands for the arms of the chair before sitting down. If she is working from the side, the nurse can place a foot behind the chair leg so that it cannot slide away.

Many patients need to relieve themselves when they first get out of bed and it is convenient for the nurse to help them directly on to the commode or sanitary chair.

Helping the patient back to bed

To get the patient back to bed the procedures are reversed. The bed should, as before, be in the low position and the wheels braked. The patient is helped to his feet, and turned round until he can sit on the edge of the bed, well up towards the pillow. If he cannot do it himself, his feet and legs are lifted on to the bed by the nurse while she supports his back.

Bed aid

Movement in and out of bed is made easier for some patients by the Economic Bed Aid (Kimberley Bingham & Co.). This is a hand rail which clamps to the bed. It can be locked into any convenient position (Fig. 26a).

Less obtrusive and perhaps more convenient is the Masterpeace lift aid. This too clamps to the side of the bed but has no moving parts (Fig. 26b). It is particularly useful at home.

Lifting belts

Some nurses find it easier to transfer a patient if he is wearing a belt. A lifting belt provides the nurse with a convenient hand hold when she is helping a patient to sit, stand, pivot or transfer.

Hoists

Adjustable height beds obviate a great deal of lifting as long as the patient can stand, taking his own weight. If he cannot and is heavy and helpless it is better to use a hoist. There are a number of types available and the nurse should know something of them.

Mobile Hydraulic Hoist

The hydraulic hoist consists of a vertical mast with a boom from which the patient is suspended in a sling. The apparatus is mounted on a mobile base, the spread of which can be adapted to pass through narrow doorways or to open out around wheelchairs and baths. These hoists need room for manoeuvring and if carelessly used can be tipped over. Space for storage may be a problem.

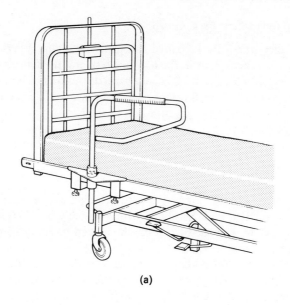

(a)

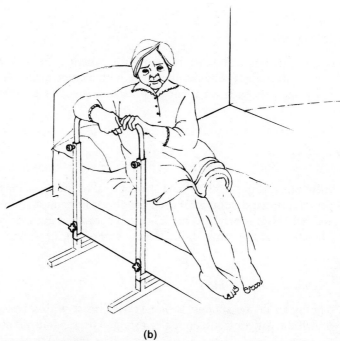

(b)

Fig. 26 Bed aids
  (a) Economic bed aid
  (b) Masterpeace lift aid

Band slings

Hoists are used with a variety of slings. A simple pair of band slings is the easiest to manage and the most comfortable models are padded. The longer sling goes under the patient's thighs and the shorter one round his back. It is important that the tension should fall first on the patient's back. In this way he will be suspended in a comfortable sitting position (Fig. 27). If the leg sling tightens first he will tip backwards and this is disturbing and dangerous. Sometimes the back sling causes pain under the axilla, particularly if the patient has an arthritic shoulder. If the patient is moved whilst suspended from a hydraulic hoist he will swing a little and this may be unnerving to him. The New Steel Nurse, a hoist invented in Holland, has a special padded harness and spreader bar which stops the patient swinging.

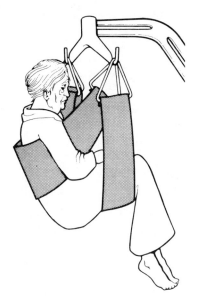

Fig. 27 Band slings

Hammock slings

A patient with a weak back may feel safer in a hammock sling. Suspended by hooks from a spreader bar it supports the whole of the back and prevents jack-knifing. Some hammock slings are now made in a one piece rectangular design with a commode aperture cut out of it (Fig. 28a). But those with divided legs are generally

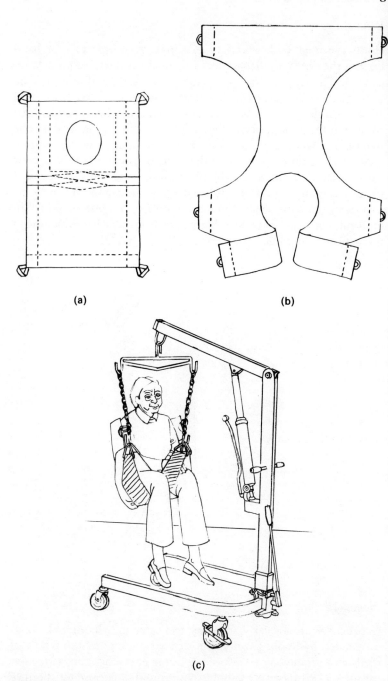

(a)

(b)

(c)

Fig. 28 a, b, c

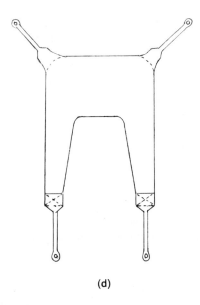

(d)

Fig. 28 Hammock slings
    (a) One piece rectangular Hammock sling with commode aperture
    (b) Hammock sling with divided legs
    (c) Hammock sling with crossed leg pieces
    (d) Easi-Use commode sling

more useful (Fig. 28b). The leg pieces may be used in one of three ways.

For toilet purposes the most obvious way is to fasten each sling round one leg. But this can be embarrassing for the patient because the legs fall apart when he is lifted.

The lift is more comfortable and dignified if the patient's legs can be held together. This is achieved by passing both slings under both thighs and fastening them to the opposite sides. This method preserves the patient's dignity, but it may make toileting more difficult.

A compromise may be achieved by passing each band under one thigh and fastening it to the opposite side. This enables the legs to be held together when the patient is lifted while providing enough separation for toileting (Fig. 28c).

FML Easi-Use commode sling

Most hammock slings require side suspenders and chains to adjust the height and allow the patient to be supported in comfort. All this is rather complicated for the nurse and the FML Easi-Use commode sling which does not require chains and can be hooked directly to the spreader bar is the easiest to understand. It is designed to go with a Commodore hoist (Fig. 28d).

Its disadvantage is that three sizes are required if all patients are to be accommodated, but it is still recommended as the most convenient hammock sling.

The Mecanaids ambulift

The ambulift is the most generally useful mobile hoist. It is popular with patients because it gives them a sense of security and with nurses because it is so versatile. The main feature is a mechanically operated hoist with detachable lightweight seat (Fig. 29a). The seat has convenient foldaway arms and a leg rest can

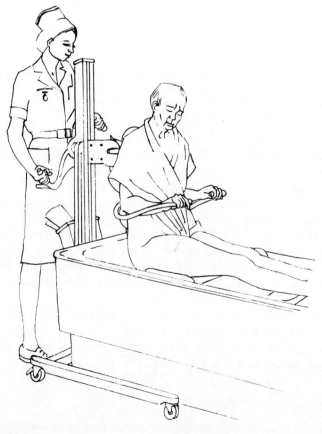

Fig. 29 a

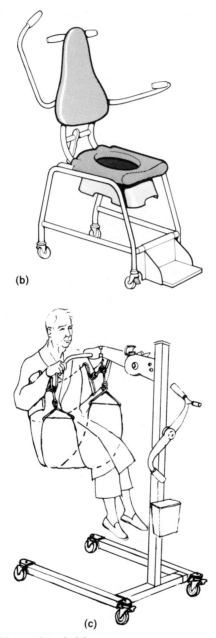

Fig. 29 The Mecanaids ambulift
    (a) Mecanaids ambulift and raised bath with recessed base
    (b) Ambulift seat attached to sub chassis becomes a sanitary chair
    (c) The ambulift adapted for use with slings

be added for additional security. Detached from the hoist and fixed to a special subchassis the seat becomes a wheelchair and can be used as a sanitary chair to take the patient to the toilet or as a shower chair to take him to the bath.

Although the ambulift was originally designed to transport the patient with the chair attached to the hoist it is generally more convenient and acceptable to the patient to use the chair and subchassis as a wheelchair. Less space is required around the bed if the hoist is left in the bathroom and only the wheelchair is brought to the bedside (Fig. 29b).

If it is decided to use the ambulift exclusively as a bathing aid there may be an advantage in using a floor mounted model which can stand at the end, side or corner of the bath. This sacrifices the mobility of the ambulift but may be very convenient if space is restricted. By adding a pan the wheelchair can become a commode.

If it is desired to exploit the full versatility of the ambulift and to use it for the patient who must be lifted bodily from his bed or chair the seat can be removed and replaced with slings. The ambulift is then used like the sling hoists already described (Fig. 29c). Alternatively for the patient in bed, the seat can be placed across the bed and the patient is assisted to roll into it. After he is seated the arms are folded into position and the ambulift is attached to the chair. The chair can then be converted into a wheelchair or the patient may be transferred in the chair attached to the mast.

There is much for the nurse to learn about the ambulift but once she has confidence in it she will discover that it is invaluable.

The Arjo Bath Hoist

The ambulift, although capable of lifting a patient from his bed, is primarily designed to take him from his chair and to lower him into the water from the end of the bath. The subchassis provides a convenient toilet chair.

In contrast the Swedish Arjo Bath Hoist is designed to take a patient to the bath from his bed, lowering him into the water from the side. To accommodate the feet of the hoist part of the bath's side panel must be cut away. The system is very convenient for bathing and can also be used to lift a patient while bed linen is changed. Its limitation is in the toilet, as the patient has to sit side-ways across the lavatory instead of in the usual position (Fig. 30).

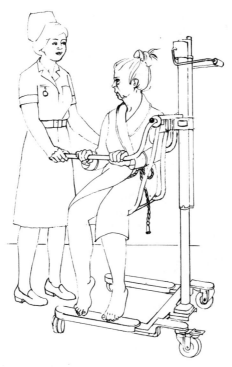

Fig. 30 The Arjo Bath Hoist

Electric gantry hoists

An electric hoist attached to an overhead gantry provides a most useful method of assisting a patient who cannot help himself in and out of bed. It is obligatory if he is on a water bed (see p. 188). In hospital the rail may be fixed to the ceiling or it may be suspended on a pair of steel supports (Fig. 31). The motor is attached to a trolley running along the rail. Any form of sling can be used with this apparatus. The standard length of rail is sufficient to span a bed, a chair and a commode placed side by side. The electric motor has many advantages (until it breaks down) and the patient may be able to operate it himself. A gantry hoist may be dismantled and erected over any bed but in a ward where space is restricted there are usually only one or two beds where a gantry hoist will fit easily. Because they are fixed they are useful only to lift a patient in and out of bed and cannot be used to take him to the bathroom or the lavatory. But for the patient whose main need is to be lifted in and out of bed the electric gantry hoist is invaluable. Its most serious disadvantage is the noise of the motor, which can be disturbing at night.

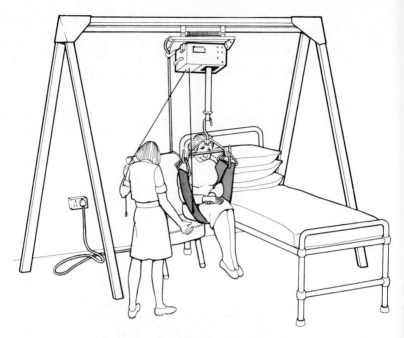

Fig. 31 Electric Gantry Hoist

Lifting in the home

All the hoists so far described may be employed in the patient's home but restricted space and low ceilings sometimes preclude their use. There are three small mobile sling hoists, the Mecanaid's Mecalift, Carter's Medi-hoist and Payne's Isis. They are mechanically, not hydraulically, operated. They come apart easily and can be carried in the boot of a car. Each is valuable for short-term use because no installation is required and the nurse can carry the apparatus to the house herself. They are of value for long-term use when a mobile rather than a static hoist is required. They will negotiate conventional doorways and narrow corridors without difficulty. The Mecalift has a device which helps it over carpets and thresholds.

For further reading:

TARLING, C. 1980. *Hoists and Their Use*. London: Heinemann.

TROUP, D., LLOYD, P., OSBORNE, C. & TARLING, C. 1981. *The Handling of Patients: A Guide for Nurse Managers*. Back Pain Association and Royal College of Nursing.

14
Furniture

The ward furniture, particularly the bed, the chair and the locker, make a most important contribution to the older patient's care. They are essential tools in rehabilitation.

The bed

A bed should of course be comfortable but the patient must be able to get in and out of it easily. At home the bed is often too low but it can be raised on blocks. In hospital it is likely to be too high. The best bed for an elderly patient who needs nursing is one of adjustable height within a range of 45 – 90 cm (18 – 36 in) from the floor to the top of the mattress. A high bed is convenient for nursing procedures and bedmaking. A low one enables the older patient to get in and out safely. The right height for any individual is one which enables him to sit on the edge of the bed with his feet flat on the floor.

Kings Fund bed

The Kings Fund design is by far the best (Fig. 32). The mechanism is foot operated and easy for the nurse to use. It has good brakes, a built-in back rest and a bed stripper. It will tilt and there are facilities for the attachment of drip stands and a lifting pole. The bed has a firm base designed to take a foam mattress. One problem with adjustable height beds is that it is possible for the head of the bed to jam against the window ledge or a wall fitting. If a bed proves difficult to raise this cause should be excluded.

Hinged bed

To sit up on a flat base imposes a shearing strain on the buttocks which can predispose to pressure sores. To offset this some modern beds have a hinged base with three or four sections. The four-section models are best and have long been popular in Scandinavia. The

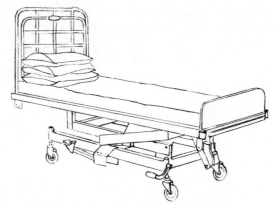

Fig. 32 Kings Fund Bed

head end can be raised to form a back rest and the middle section gives support behind the thighs. Electrical operation is available but adds to the cost. One disadvantage of hinged beds is that men find it difficult to use a urinal when the bed is in the hinged position.

Mattress

The conventional polyurethane foam mattress has not proved durable and when covered with a waterproof sheet does not allow sufficient ventilation. The Vaperm mattress has been specially designed to overcome these defects. It has firm plastic foam at the edges of the mattress and softer foam in the centre. It is covered by a waterproof but vapour permeable material. It may well prove to be the mattress of the future.

Bedding

When the patient is in bed, his comfort is all important and tidiness is of secondary consideration. In hospital, sheets and cellular blankets made of cotton are almost universally used because they can be boiled in the laundry which reduces the risk of cross infection. At home, however, the top blankets may be replaced by a duvet or continental quilt provided it is fire resistant. Duvets are light and warm and reduce the work of bed making. They are particularly appreciated by arthritic patients. Duvets were at first suitable only for continent patients, but their use is increasing since the introduction of the Belmont duvet (Lackworth Medical Products). This has a ventilated and welded PVC cover which can be wiped clean as often as is necessary. The material is comfortable enough to wear against the skin. A detachable cover of fire retardant material is an optional extra and is all that need be sent to the laundry.

Sheepskins

Natural sheepskins are very comfortable to sit on. They offer good ventilation to the buttocks and heels, absorb moisture and probably contribute to the prevention of pressure sores. They do not, however, stand up well to frequent laundering and so are unsuitable for the incontinent. Synthetic pads are less absorbent and to this extent less comforting but they are cheaper, easier to launder and have a long life even when used for incontinent patients. In hospital their best use is for patients in long-stay wards, particularly those who are not incontinent. Their main use, however, is probably for patients nursed at home. A new development for home use is the artificial sheepskin used as a fitted underblanket.

Draw sheets

Draw sheets have maintained their place as part of hospital equipment ever since they were introduced in the 19th century as a way to save linen. If the patient is continent there is no need for a draw sheet. Where there is a risk that the patient will be incontinent a draw sheet with a layer of polythene underneath it may be used in the traditional position across the bed. An alternative which some nurses favour is to put the draw sheet longwise in the bed, again with a layer of polythene underneath it.

Safety sides

The old fashioned cot bed is now obsolete but a few patients, probably not more than one or two in any ward, need safety sides. The most convenient are those which are permanently attached to the bed and can be hinged upwards for use when required.

The proper use of safety sides is to protect the patient who is in danger of falling out of bed through physical infirmity. Some patients, especially the blind, find safety sides reassuring. Others, for example, hemiplegics can move in bed more freely if they grasp the bars with their one good hand. Safety sides should not run the full length of the bed but, as in the ship's bunk, should be used to give a feeling of security rather than imprisonment and the best models are now of adjustable length. The bars should be close enough together to prevent the patient getting his head stuck between them.

There is a temptation to use safety sides to restrain the restless patient. This is not good practice. To leave a patient caged behind bars may cause him much distress and perhaps provoke incontinence. He may well want to go to the lavatory, although unable to express his wishes except perhaps by rattling the bars. It is better for such a patient if the nurse ensures that the bed is in the low position, and is prepared to assist him to his feet and to discover where he wants to go. A restless patient with enough determination will climb over any safety side but he risks a serious fall in doing so.

Bed tables

A suitable bed table plays a large part in the patient's comfort. A cantilever table of adjustable height and angle is best. These tables serve equally well for the patient in bed or in a chair. They are light and easy to move. The more expensive models also contain a small drawer with a collapsible mirror and book rest.

The bedside locker

The older patient needs his clothes with him when he is in hospital. In some hospitals clothes are kept in individual cupboards and the patient has a conventional bedside locker. Most nurses agree that it is preferable for the patient to have a wardrobe locker so that he has the security of knowing that his belongings are right beside his bed. The St. Helen's wardrobe locker is suitable (Fig. 33a). It provides sufficient drawer and hanging space and has room for a mirror and a towel rail. The unit can be built with the wardrobe to the right or the left of the locker so that it can stand on either side of the bed but it cannot conveniently go on the 'wrong' side. The Hoskins Arden locker is different. This locker can be turned so that the locker is in front of the wardrobe which can then be opened from either side. Or it can be used in the conventional way with a locker and the wardrobe side by side (Fig. 33b). Lockers are now made in attractive colours which, if the ward has a variety, can be used to individualise the patient's bed space.

The chair

It is important to have a variety of chairs in a ward for the elderly. As well as armchairs there must be plenty of dining chairs placed

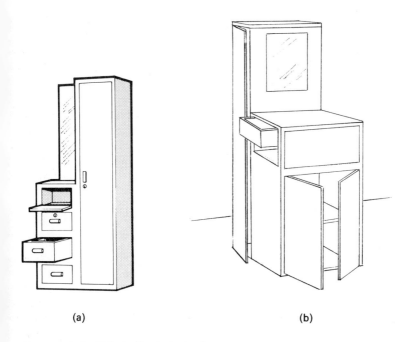

(a)   (b)

Fig. 33 (a) St. Helen's Wardrobe Locker
(b) Hoskins Arden Locker

round tables for meals and other activities. In general the chair for the older patient should be easy to get in and out of, sufficiently high to make it easy to rise but low enough for the patient's feet to rest firmly on the floor. These requirements are usually met by a chair whose seat is about 46 cm (18 in) from the floor, but any ward should contain a selection with seats from 40 to 55 cm (16–22 in). Some of the most useful chairs are of adjustable height. The arms should come well forward but not so far that the chair tips up when the patient pushes himself to his feet. Some models have dropped hand rests (Fig. 34a). Equally the chair must not tip sideways when the patient puts all his weight on one arm as he may do if he is hemiplegic. There should be no rail between the front legs because this prevents the patient tucking his feet back under the chair when rising. The back should be high enough to support the head and shoulders with a bulge in the lumbar region. There should be no gap between the back and the seat. Wings may be useful for some patients whose heads need additional support but they tend to isolate the patient from his neighbours by making conversation more difficult.

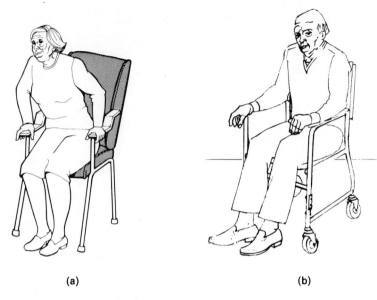

(a)   **(b)**

Fig. 34 (a) Dining chair with lowered handrests
(b) Glideabout chair

Mobile 'geriatric' chairs

Since the aim for most patients is rehabilitation the majority of
chairs for use both in the day area and at the bedside should be of the
static type. But there is a need for some mobile 'geriatric' chairs for
the most feeble patients, particularly in long-stay units.

Mobile 'geriatric' chairs are usually fitted with a detachable tray.
This may be appropriate for the very frail but more independent
individuals may feel affronted or imprisoned by it. It is usually better
to sit the patient at a table. It is not good practice to use a tray as a
restraint. If the patient is restless in a chair it may be better to take
him for a walk.

Transit chairs

Mobile 'geriatric' chairs can be used to take a patient from his
bedside to the day room but it is usually better to use a small transit
chair, such as a glideabout or a model 9 (Fig. 34b) with four small
wheels. It is more work for the nurse to help a patient from his
bedside chair into a transit chair and again from the transit chair into
a static chair in the day room but each movement is a valuable form

of physiotherapy, contributes to his rehabilitation and diminishes the risk of pressure sores.

There is a need for suitable wheelchairs for patients who can be taken out of doors into a garden or on outings. Chairs for this purpose should be folding so that they can be placed in the boot of a car.

Self-propelling wheelchairs are of limited use in departments of medicine for the elderly. If required they should be prescribed by the occupational therapist in conjunction with the representative of the Department of Health and Social Security wheelchair centre. A selection of types should be available in a central point such as the occupational therapy department. Only a patient's personal wheel-chair should be kept on the wards.

Ejector chairs and seats

Ejector chairs and seats have become much less widely used since the introduction of adjustable height chairs. The only indication for an ejector chair is if it enables a patient to get up from a chair when he cannot do so from one of adjustable height even when it has been raised.

Tables

An increasingly important part of the older patient's day should be spent sitting at a table for occupational therapy, diversional activity, meals or conversation. It is not only more like normal life to eat and work at a table in company with others but the effort of moving there in itself provides purposeful activity and encourages walking.

Chairs and tables must be considered together. Chairs with arms are more suitable for the older patient but the arms must fit under the table. Square or rectangular tables with legs at the corners are more suitable than pedestal tables which are less secure. The best height is 71 cm (28 in). In occupational therapy departments an adjustable height table has proved of value. The table top should not be more than 5 cm thick (2 in) so as to leave room for the chair arms.

Ward safety

To keep the patient out of bed, to encourage him to dress, to walk to the toilet, to do as much as possible for himself inevitably exposes him to risks. Regrettably, minor accidents and occasionally more serious ones happen even in the best departments. They must be regarded as the price to be paid for the improved quality of life which a policy of activation brings. It is very seldom justified to restrain an old person to prevent an accident. The nurse must feel confident that her managers will support her if an accident occurs when she has done her best.

Accidents are less likely if the ward is properly equipped. Observation is easier in an old fashioned Nightingale ward, but modern wards with six-bedded bays have so many other advantages that they are preferred. Many falls occur when a patient is getting up or going to bed. It is important that there should be adequate space in the bed area so that the nurse can help the patient without having to move the furniture. About 6 sq m cubicle space or 2.7 m (9 ft) between bed centres should suffice. There should be a non-slip rug by each bed unless the floor is carpeted.

Adjustable height beds should normally be in the low position to enable the patient to get in and out safely. Their wheels should always be braked, as should those of commodes and wheelchairs whenever the patient is transferring.

Baths, toilets and the passages leading to them must be well lit and equipped with suitable handrails (see p. 220). Stairs must have a rail on each side.

Accidents are most likely when ward activity is greatest and the nurse is unable to give her undivided attention to any one patient. If patient activity can be staggered, so that, for example, not everyone is attempting to dress at the same time, the atmosphere will be calmer and the patient will feel more secure. Falls are less likely when the patient is allowed to take his time. The best insurance is a team of well trained nurses who plan their work carefully.

For further reading:

COAKLEY, D. (Ed). 1982. *Establishing a Geriatric Service* (Chapter 6). Beckenham: Croom Helm.

HARRIS, C. & MAYFIELD, W. 1983. *Selecting Easy Chairs for Elderly and Disabled People*. Institute for Consumer Ergonomics, University of Technology, Loughborough.

TUDOR, M. A. 1981. *A Wheelchair Is Requested*. Royal Home and Hospital for Incurables (RHHI Publications).

15
Cleanliness and Skin Care

Cleanliness makes an important contribution to comfort but washing is an individual affair and potentially embarrassing to the older patient. It is one of the few occasions in life when a person is exposed naked to a stranger who may be of the opposite sex. It therefore requires sensitivity on the part of the nurse.

People vary greatly in their habits. To some a bath is a daily necessity, to others an unfamiliar ordeal. As far as resources permit the patient should be allowed to choose how often he takes a bath.

Bed baths

The acutely ill or terminal patient needs a bed bath each day. The nurse should try to follow the patient's wishes, for example in the matter of soap on his face or the use of talcum powder. As always, she will encourage him to do anything he can for himself. Even bed bathing can contribute to a patient's rehabilitation. If he has a hemiplegia, for example, the nurse must move the arm to wash the axilla. In so doing she is performing a useful bit of physiotherapy.

Sometimes bed bathing involves two nurses. If so they should resist the temptation to talk to one another across the patient and make an effort to bring him into any conversation.

In the bathroom

Bed bathing is only for the very ill. It is preferable to use the bathroom whenever possible, particularly for those with stiff joints, who are helped by lying in hot water. The room should be warm, the window shut and the floor dry. The patient should be offered the toilet before he goes to the bathroom. The nurse fills the bath and checks the temperature. The proper temperature is one which is comfortable for the patient's feet, normally the coldest part of the body. If the patient has a dry skin or likes the scent, bath oil may be added to the water but it will make the bath more slippery.

Aids to bathing

Most old people are capable of bathing themselves but are safer if the bathroom is properly equipped. The bath needs a non-slip surface. This can be provided by self-adhesive non-slip strips or a rubber mat with multiple small suction cups on the underside. The mat should lie under the patient's legs so that it is in the right position when he stands up. Mats adhere best when the bath is wet. They must be pushed down firmly to make the suckers grip.

If a patient can step over the side of the bath he will be more secure if there is something to grasp. A simple upright pole from floor to ceiling or a rail clamped onto the side of the bath are both suitable. They should be placed about 40 cm (16 in) from the taps (Fig. 35a). Alternatively an 'Economic Bath Aid' may be used. This is fixed to the taps and spans the bath. It is rather low for someone getting into the bath but useful to pull on when he is getting out. It is hinged and can be folded out of the way when not required. If the bath is placed against the wall some form of wall mounted handrail is useful. This can be horizontal, vertical or sloping (Fig. 35).

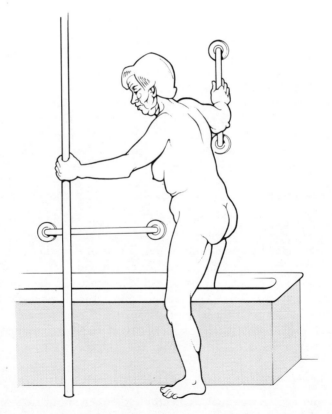

Fig. 35 a

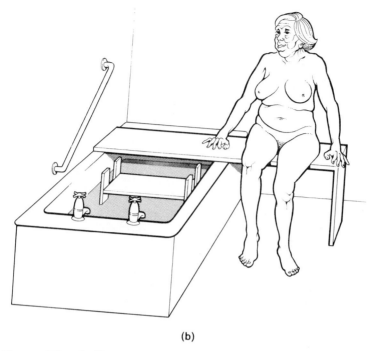

(b)

Fig. 35 Aids to bathing
  (a) Upright pole and wall mounted bath rails
  (b) Bath bridge, bath seat and wall mounted sloping rail

It is easier to get up from a sitting position, so many old people like a bath seat. The wooden type which wedges into the bath is the safest. Many geriatric day hospitals make them in their workshops. The bath seat may be used with a bath bridge. This spans the bath, extending about 250 mm (10 in) over the side. It enables the patient to slide over the bath before lowering himself onto the seat or into the water. A rail sloping downwards and forwards from the back of the bath gives additional safety (Fig. 35b). If a bath bridge is used a full sized bath is necessary. Otherwise a shorter bath, about 1.5 m long, is safer and easier to get out of.

The Autolift. A sophisticated aid which enables the patient who cannot step or slide into the bath is the Autolift (Mecanaids Ltd.). The patient sits in a chair which is attached to a column fixed to the floor beside the bath. Within the column is a hand operated lifting mechanism. Its handle can be used by the patient himself or by the nurse (Fig. 36).

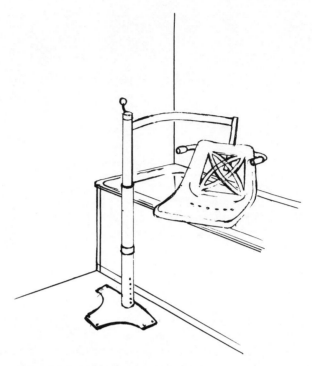

Fig. 36 Mecanaids floor mounted Autolift

Types of bath

No one bath is suitable for all purposes. A well equipped ward needs a selection.

There should be at least one conventional bath so that a patient who is capable of doing so can bath himself in the ordinary way with such aids as are necessary.

The patient who must be bathed by an attendant should use a raised bath to spare the nurse's back. The patient is lifted in and out by a hoist (see pp. 150–3). The most convenient height for a raised bath is 850 mm (33 in).

If a mobile hoist is to be used the side panels of the bath must be recessed to allow room for its feet (see Fig. 29a). If a static hoist is fixed by the side of the bath, a recessed base may still be convenient for the nurse's toes.

Adjustable height bath. If space is at a premium and there is room for only one bath an adjustable height bath is a solution, though expensive (Fig. 37).

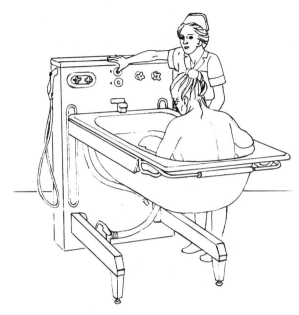

Fig. 37 Mecanaids adjustable height bath

In the low position it can be used as a standard bath by the patient who can do things for himself. With the bath in the high position and using an ambulift the nurse can bathe her more dependent patients.

The Parker bath. An important development in bath equipment which avoids the need for a hoist is the height adjustable and tilting Parker bath. This won the Prince of Wales Award for Industrial Innovation in 1982.

The bath is mounted on a pedestal and tilts backwards like a dentist's chair. It has a foot well and a seat. There is a hinged side panel, which lifts up out of the way, allowing the user to enter by sitting on the seat and lifting his legs in after him. The foot well is filled with warm water before the patient gets in (Fig. 38a). The side panel is lowered to form a watertight seal. The bath is then tilted so that the patient lies in a reclining position and the water flows around him (Fig. 38b). To get out of the bath the patient or the nurse operates a release mechanism which restores the bath to the upright position. The side panel is lifted out of the way and the patient steps or slides out. He can be partially dried before he leaves the bath.

This bath is proving increasingly popular both in hospital and in the home. It is fairly expensive but costs a good deal less than a height adjustable bath that must be used with a hoist.

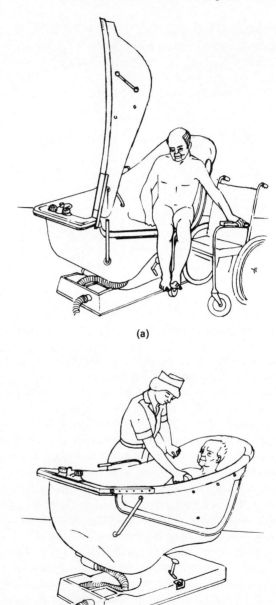

(a)

(b)

Fig. 38 The Parker Bath
    (a) Entering the Parker bath
    (b) The Parker bath in use

Medic Bath. Bathing is easier for the nurse and the patient if he can walk into the bath and wash sitting down. This is the object of the Medic Bath. It consists of a shower cabinet 914 mm (36 in) deep and 864 mm (34 in) high with a removable front panel. The patient steps in over a low sill, turns round and sits down using the sides for support. The front panel is then replaced and the patient is washed with a hand spray.

For those who cannot step over the raised sill there is a detachable ramp to assist entry. The Medic Bath can also be fitted with an optional sliding seat for the more disabled.

Where space is restricted this bath is useful and some people are enthusiastic about its virtues.

Shower

In most parts of the world showers are the standard method of bathing and in Britain they are gaining wider acceptance. With proper facilities a shower is quicker, more hygienic and more economic of water than any other way of bathing.

The most disabled patient can use a shower provided he does not have to negotiate a step. This rules out the conventional shower cubicle and means that the shower room must be purpose built, with its floor flush to the rest of the bathroom and with a drain in the middle (Fig. 39). The design should include a curtained changing area at the entrance where the patient can undress and the nurse don her waterproofs.

Most old people should shower sitting down. They can enter by sliding along a fixed bench with appropriate handrails or in a mobile shower chair which should have a brake. The ambulift seat attached to its subchassis makes an excellent shower chair for the patient who has been faecally incontinent. For the occasional patient who prefers to shower standing up there must be suitably placed handrails, a non-slip mat and a built-in soap dish.

Showering should always be done with a hand set. The patient should never be deluged from a fixed spray above his head. The temperature of the water should be regulated thermostatically and the shower and changing areas must be comfortably warm.

Washing

Regular washing of the face and hands contributes as much to the comfort of the older patient as does his bath. If possible he should wash himself at a basin, do his own hair, shave himself with an

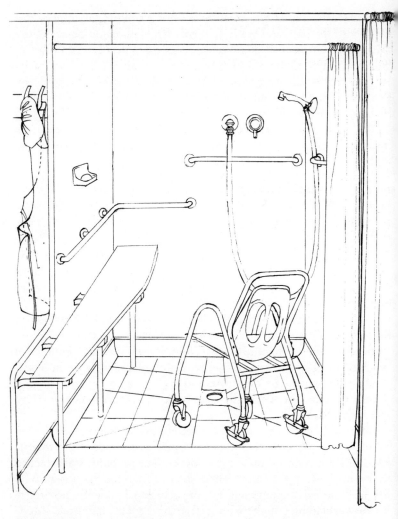

Fig. 39 Shower room. Note changing area, bench with handrail, shower chair, flexible hand set and level floor with drain

electric razor and clean his own teeth. If he can do these things for himself the nurse should resist the temptation to help him in order to save time. To do something for the patient that he can do for himself is to rob him of his independence.

Some patients need to wash in bed. The bowl is placed on a cantilever table together with the washing things. The bedside locker is not a suitable place for a bowl. It is too far behind the patient when he sits up in bed. There are other patients, however, who like to dress sitting on the side of the bed and to wash before they do so. For them the bedside locker is a convenient place for the bowl.

Patients normally wash in the ward night and morning but they will want other opportunities to wash their hands when they are in the day room, before meals and after they have been to the toilet. Ill patients who are confined to bed may appreciate the opportunity to freshen up with a medicated wipe.

Mouth hygiene

Mouth hygiene is important for the older patient. A dirty mouth may be cleaned with bicarbonate swabs and special attention should be paid to food which may have lodged in the paralysed cheek of the patient with hemiplegia. Afterwards the patient should be offered a thymol mouthwash, but if he is confused and likely to swallow the mouthwash, plain water is better. To finish with a lemon and glycerine swab will leave the patient refreshed.

A dry mouth may be due to drugs, particularly anti-depressants and anti-spasmodics. It may be due to mouth breathing, but an important factor is usually dehydration. The best prevention is to give sufficient fluid.

A sore mouth may be due to stomatitis, ulceration or to thrush. Thrush will respond to Nystatin suspension, Fungilin lozenges or Daktarin Oral Gel.

Teeth

A patient who can wash himself can usually brush his own teeth and should be given the opportunity to do so. Dentures should be cleaned at least once a day though after every meal is the ideal. They should be held under running water and brushed with a denture brush. A denture powder can be used if desired. There should be some water in the wash basin. If the denture is dropped it will fall into water and is less likely to break. While the denture is being cleaned the patient can be offered a mouth wash. Some people prefer to omit the brushing and simply sprinkle the denture with powder, leaving it in water over night. A supply of fixative should be available for those with loose dentures. If this does not solve the problem the dentist may advise relining.

Dentures should be marked as soon as possible after the patient's admission to the ward. They are easily lost or mixed up and may then be impossible to identify. The Identure marking system is very satisfactory. The area of denture to be marked is cleaned with one of the small pads provided. The denture is then marked with a felt tipped pen which writes in grey or black as required. The ink is then covered by two coats of sealing liquid. The whole procedure takes only a few minutes.

Hair

The patient's hair should be brushed and combed twice a day and tidied when necessary. It should be washed every week if possible. An attractive hair style is a morale booster at any age and the nurse should take pains to help her patients look their best. No woman is too old to enjoy a hair-do but many old people cannot get to a hairdresser. In hospital a professional hairdresser should visit the wards regularly and many patients will be glad to pay for her services. Every women's ward should have hairdryers. The hood type is most generally useful but for the very frail patient who cannot hold her head up a hand held model is necessary.

Makeup and manicure

Most women should be encouraged to use their normal cosmetics. Some patients, especially those in long-stay units, benefit from the beauty therapy and manicure services offered by the British Red Cross.

Although modern bedside lockers incorporate a mirror it is not always well placed for the patient to use from his bed. A shaving or makeup mirror is a useful accessory.

Nails

The patient's nails should be kept clean and cut every week. The best time is after a bath when they are softened by hot water. Toe nails should be trimmed straight across to prevent ingrowing. They are not always easy to cut without nail clippers. Careless or inexpert nail cutting may lead to gangrene in people with poor peripheral circulation. Such patients, especially if diabetic, should be treated by a chiropodist.

Pressure areas

The care of pressure areas is an important part of nursing, particularly in old age when the skin loses some of its suppleness. In the past attention has been paid not only to frequent washing of the skin, especially when there is incontinence, but also to its medication. The nurse has been advised to rub in soap, spirit, witch-hazel and the like. Research has shown, however, that all these practices are harmful. Spirit removes sebum, the skin's natural lubrication, while too much soap, which is strongly alkaline, alters the skin's pH rendering it more permeable and can leave irritant deposits. Even rubbing alone may damage the microcirculation and increase the risk of sores.

A daily wash of the pressure areas with soap and water is beneficial and hygienic but when more frequent washes are needed, as with incontinent patients, the nurse is advised to use plenty of water but only the minimum of soap and to rinse it off well.

Innumerable preparations have been advocated for the protection of the skin but there is little to choose between them and many have disadvantages. Barrier creams, for example, protect the skin from external irritants but they also protect it from air which prevents moisture from evaporating and leaves the skin soggy. Two of the best and cheapest preparations for local application are zinc cream and arachis oil.

Spray preparations are convenient but more expensive. Because the nurse does not have to touch the patient's skin when using them it is said that there is a reduced risk of cross infection. This is probably a rather theoretical advantage but the sprays are certainly handy.

In the Hastings Department of Medicine for the Elderly no local application is used routinely unless the patient is incontinent when benzalkonium and cetrimide cream, Drapolene, is applied if there is a urine rash. The most important elements in the preservation of the skin are the regular relief of pressure and adequate ventilation.

Protection of the heels

The heels are vulnerable in the older patient and need careful protection. The patient with a fractured femur or a hemiplegia is at special risk. By far the most important measure is the use of a cantilever bed cradle to take the weight of the bedclothes and to permit free movement. A cantilever cradle should be put in from the end of the bed with the longer portion under the mattress. It is less satisfactory to put it in from the side as the patient may strike his feet against it. A properly equipped acute ward should have a cradle to every bed but not all patients will welcome this. Some will say that they cannot get their feet warm. This is one of the few times that the nurse must be insistent. The patient can, however, have a light cellular blanket next to him if he wishes.

In convalescent and continuing care wards there is little risk of pressure sores and cradles need not be used unless the patient becomes acutely ill again. When bed cradles are needed only occasionally, a folding model is more convenient if there are problems of storage. When no cradle is used the nurse must be careful to leave some slack in the bedclothes to allow freedom of movement. If the patient is in bed when it is made he can be asked to cross his legs before the blankets are tucked in.

Efforts may also be made to protect the heels directly. The old fashioned heel ring is obsolete as it merely transfers the pressure from one small area to another. A tubipad (an elasticated tubular bandage incorporating a strip of plastic foam), which should be worn next to the skin, is disposable and cheap, and has been popular for many years. It is important to ensure that the padding is placed to protect the points of pressure when the patient is turned. The tubipad should extend to the patient's toes or the forefoot may swell.

Bootees with natural or synthetic sheepskin are more expensive but they cover the malleoli as well as the heels. They are more comfortable and probably more effective. A useful compromise may be the elastic tubular bandage incorporating a sheepskin lining, e.g. the Seaton parapad which has proved very acceptable.

An important new development is the Spenco foot pillow. These are made from synthetic fibre coated with silicone and feel like a soft feather bed. They support the entire foot and are washable.

The heel on which a sore is threatening may be lifted off the bed by resting the leg on a wedge of plastic foam, the Lennard pad, or on a bead filled cushion.

Protection of the buttocks

The patient who sits for long periods in a chair is at risk for pressure sores over the ischial tuberosities. The best preventative is the regular movement provided by trips to the toilet, but the seat on which he sits is also of importance.

A well designed armchair should have a comfortable seat and needs no more than perhaps to be covered by a sheepskin.

A patient in a wheelchair is normally provided with a foam cushion. An alternative is the Spenco cushion which is made of the same silicone material as the foot pillow described above. It is soft and comfortable. One side is covered by a material which breathes, the other with waterproof material for the patient who is incontinent (Fig. 40a). The cushion is washable in a hospital laundry. A larger size with back and sides is also available.

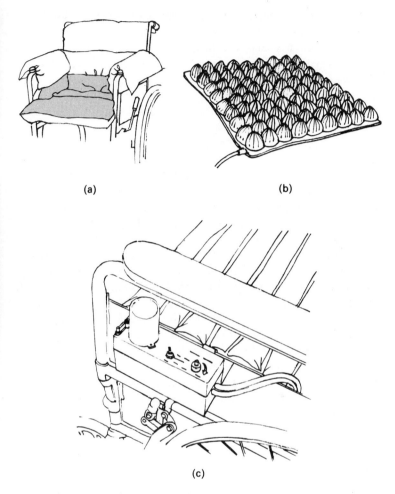

(a) (b)

(c)

Fig. 40 Pressure relieving cushions
(a) Spenco cushion
(b) Roho dry flotation cushion
(c) Ripple cushion

The Roho dry flotation cushion consists of a system of interconnected but separate air cells (Fig. 40b). The cushion is blown up like a bicycle tyre. It is usual to over-inflate it at first and let the air out gradually until the patient is comfortable. This point is usually reached when the nurse can just slide one finger underneath his ischium. The instructions supplied with the cushion should be followed carefully. The manufacturers offer a telephone advisory service on 04912−78446 to any patient who feels he is not getting the best out of his cushion.

Gel cushions are made of a material with a consistency similar to that of human fat. They are usually very heavy and feel cold when the patient first sits on them but their pressure relieving properties are good.

A number of cushions combine water and foam, for example the Dyson cushion (Huntleigh) and the Hydromedica flotation cushion (3M UK Ltd.). The Seabird cushion combines a gel core with an air surround (Mayflower). These cushions are really designed for a patient in a wheelchair. If placed in an armchair they tend to make the seat too high.

The position of the patient, particularly in a wheelchair, is of importance. If he sits with his thighs parallel to the floor his weight will be distributed between his buttocks and his thighs. If the leg rests are too high and the patient tilts backwards more weight will be taken on the buttocks. If the arm rests are of an appropriate height some weight can be taken periodically by the arms which relieves the buttocks.

A person who sits with a tilted pelvis, the result perhaps of a stiff hip or curvature of the spine, may need special support to avoid taking too much weight on one side.

An alternative way of relieving pressure, appropriate to both armchairs and wheelchairs, is the ripple cushion which has been available for many years (Fig. 40c). It works on the same principle as the ripple mattress (see p. 182). The motor is driven by a rechargeable battery attached to the chair. Since the battery has a limited life it is important that it should be recharged every night.

For further reading:

TORRANCE, C. 1983. *Pressure Sores: Aetiology, Treatment and Prevention*. Beckenham: Croom Helm.

16
Pressure Sores

Pressure sores occur almost entirely in those who are ill and immobile. About 3 per cent of patients in a general hospital and
considerably more in the acute wards of a geriatric unit are affected.
Almost all sores occur within a short time of the patient's admission
to hospital. They are of two types.

Superficial sores

Superficial sores are partial thickness lesions, affecting only the
skin itself. The underlying tissues are not involved. The sores begin
as a superficial area of erythema and may develop no further. If the
situation is not relieved the erythema is succeeded within a day or
two by blistering and this may break down to leave a painful shallow
ulcer. The general condition of the patient is not affected.

Pressure is the principal factor in the development of these sores.
Its relief remains all important, but other factors contribute also.
These include abrasions from rough sheets and careless lifting, and in
the incontinent, irritation of the skin by ammonia released from the
urine. Provided pressure is relieved and they are kept clean,
superficial sores heal readily, with or without a dressing. Even in
incontinent patients the sore will heal if pressure is relieved.

Urine rash

A urine rash in an incontinent patient with poorly ventilated skin
looks rather like a superficial pressure sore, but it is more diffuse. A
pressure sore is localised over bony prominences.

Deep sores

Deep sores are far more serious. They affect the full thickness of
the skin and the underlying tissues. The damage begins deeply and
works its way to the surface. They are caused by unrelieved pressure
on the skin and underlying soft tissue against the bony prominences
of the body. They occur most frequently on the back over the
sacrum, on the buttocks, over the ischia, on the hips over the

trochanters and on the heels. An additional factor is the shearing strain which occurs when an ill patient is nursed in a semi-recumbent position and keeps slipping down the bed (Fig. 41). These two factors lead to thrombosis and rupture of the deeper vessels and thus to obliteration of the blood supply. The overlying tissues, deprived of blood, begin to die and the damage rapidly extends to the surface. An indurated mass is felt in the threatened area and soon the dead skin and subcutaneous tissue form a black eschar. Eventually this separates, leaving a deep infected ulcer going down to the bone, which may itself become involved. The patient with a deep pressure sore is always in poor general condition and his prognosis bad, though mercifully he suffers little pain.

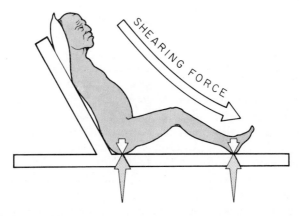

Fig. 41 Shearing force: strain is most likely to contribute to pressure sores when the patient is semi-recumbent

Healing

Sores are the result of ischaemia caused by pressure on otherwise healthy tissue. They will heal if conditions can be created which allow them to do so. This is not always true of heel sores, however, where there may be an element of peripheral vascular disease. Heel sores are four times commoner in smokers. Healing takes a long time and is sometimes incomplete.

A full thickness pressure sore heals like any other wound containing dead tissue. There are three phases.

First the dead tissue including the black slough has to liquefy and discharge. This usually takes at least two weeks. The end result should be a clean cavity.

In the second phase the surrounding skin and subcutaneous tissues contract and the wound becomes smaller.

Finally the wound cavity gradually fills with granulation tissue and eventually skin grows over it. Very big sores may fail to heal completely and surgical help may be needed to close them.

At risk patients

Normally even in sleep a person changes his position every few minutes, and thus avoids sustained pressure on any one part. Some old people when ill lose this power of spontaneous movement. They then become liable to pressure sores. The risk is greatest in those who are unconscious, paralysed or rendered immobile by traction and splints. Excessive sedation depresses bodily movement and predisposes to pressure sores, as does prolonged surgical anaesthesia. Pressure sores occur most often in bedfast patients, but those who sit too long in chairs without changing their position are also at risk.

Prevention of pressure sores

Pressure sores are distressing to the patient and may contribute to his death. They are very difficult to cure and increase greatly the amount of nursing he requires and the time he must spend in hospital. It is therefore important to make every effort to prevent them. Prevention depends on the relief of sustained pressure and shearing strain. The latter is prevented by nursing the patient flat or well propped up and not semi-recumbent. Pressure can be relieved by nursing the at risk patient in a way that distributes his weight so widely that the blood supply to the skin is not obliterated. The alternative is turning every two hours.

Two-hourly turning

Those at risk will be identified by clinical assessment or by the Norton score (see p. 72). The patient can lie for two hours on his right side, two hours on his back, two hours on his left side, provided he is conscious. If he is unconscious he must lie always on one side or the other and never on his back because of the risk that his tongue may obstruct the airway. Turning must continue at night despite the slight disturbance of the patient's rest.

Technique of turning

Turning demands two nurses who should stand one on either side of the patient's bed. If the patient is lying on his back and is to be turned on to his side, what will be his under arm is pulled a little away from his body. His upper arm is pulled across his waist, and his upper leg crossed over the other. In this way the weight of the patient's limbs can be used to assist the nurses. The nurses then place their hands on the patient's buttocks and shoulders, one pulls the upper side of the patient's body towards, the other the underside. The patient is thus turned on to his side. Once he is turned his upper knee and hip should be flexed and the underlying hip and knee extended. A pillow may be placed between his legs and another at his back on the bed or tucked under the mattress, to keep him on his side. It is also important to see that his head is comfortable.

Singlehanded turning

A nurse on her own can turn a patient easily and safely if she has the right equipment. The Norwegian Mini-Paroll, 'the nurse's third arm', fulfills this need and is particularly useful for the nurse in the community. It consists of a polished wooden board which the nurse slides under the patient's trunk and uses as a lever. The patient is secured to it by a webbing strap with a quick release buckle. Once the patient is turned the nurse can hold him in position resting the board against her shoulder, which leaves both hands free to attend to him (Fig. 42).

Mattresses

A number of special mattresses are available which contribute to the care of the patient at risk for pressure sores. Some offer intermittent relief of pressure, others distribute pressure more widely and thus reduce it over bony prominences. The best also improve the ventilation of the patient's skin. Only the most expensive remove the need for two-hourly turning.

Alternating pressure mattress (ripple bed). The alternating pressure mattress or ripple bed has been available for over twenty years. There are a number of different makes, but they all work on the same principle. They consist of an air mattress divided into cells which are slowly inflated and deflated in rotation by an electric pump (Fig. 43a and b). Most of the cells are in tubes which run

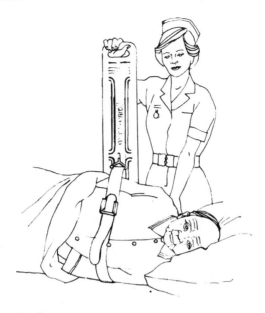

Fig. 42 Mini-Paroll

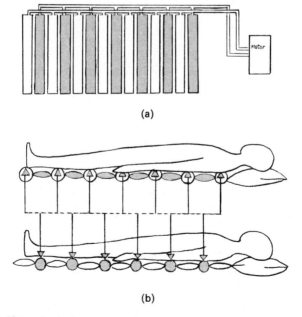

(a)

(b)

Fig. 43 Alternating pressure mattress
    (a) From above
    (b) From the side

transversely across the mattress, but there are also bubble pads in which the cells are circular. The cycle of inflation and deflation usually takes five to ten minutes. This causes a constant slight change in the distribution of the patient's weight. The large celled Ripple Mattress (Talley) is the only one proved in a controlled trial to be effective. But the Hawksley Rippling Bed, the Huntleigh Alphabed and the Mayflower Seabird mattress are probably equally effective. They are certainly all acceptable to the patient and to the nurse. The few patients who complain that alternating pressure mattresses are uncomfortable are usually those who are alert, relatively fit and not at risk for pressure sores.

Dr Mary Bliss, who has done important research on pressure sores, points out that the mattresses must be in good working order, properly installed and switched on. It is easy for the plug to be removed when someone needs the power point for another purpose. It is easy also for the tubes leading from the motor to the mattress to become kinked during bed making. It should be possible at all times to see the tubes unobstructed all the way from the mattress to the outlet nozzle of the motor.

An alternating pressure mattress which is working effectively must develop sufficient pressure to lift the patient off the bed when the cell is fully inflated. A nurse should be able to pass her arm under a deflated cell and to feel for herself that the patient is suspended above the bed. If this cannot be done the pressure setting on the dial should be checked. If the pressure is correct the mattress must be examined for faults. Any mattress in which both sets of cells are soft or hard at the same time is not working properly. The fault may lie in a tube becoming detached from the motor or from one of the cell outlet nozzles. Alternatively the fabric of a cell may be leaking. The smallest leak can prevent a mattress from working properly. Less commonly the fault lies in the motor.

The motor has a yellow light which shows that the machine is working. A large-celled mattress takes about forty-five minutes to fill with air and during this time a red light also shows on the motor. It goes out when the mattress has attained its correct pressure. A red light that remains on at any other time is a sign of danger and the cause should be investigated. Both lights go out, however, if the motor is unplugged.

In the Talley Ripple Mattress the pressure must be adjusted to the patient's weight. There is a control on the motor for this. Light patients (up to 54 kg) require a pressure of 50 mmHg. Heavy patients (over 66 kg) require 90 mmHg and medium patients between these extremes 70 mmHg.

Alternating pressure mattresses are relatively cheap to purchase but their maintenance in good working order is a problem which few hospitals have solved.

Alternating pressure mattresses with ventilation. Another problem of alternating pressure mattresses is insufficient ventilation of the patient's skin which may become macerated by urine or sweat. To overcome this there is a new generation of alternating pressure mattresses which allow air to escape from pinholes in the air cells of the mattress in order to ventilate the skin. These are the Astec AP bed and the Pegasus Airwave System (AWS) bed. An additional feature is that the alternating pressure cells rest on a static air mattress which gives extra comfort. With the Astec AP bed the nurse can vary the ripple cycle from 12 to 120 seconds. The rapid cycle provides a massaging effect to the patient's skin.

No plastic drawsheet must be used with these beds since this would obstruct the circulation of the air. But a washable fleece which is permeable to air may be used with advantage.

At present the AWS bed is available for hire from Dermalex Co. Ltd. but not for purchase. It has been shown in a controlled trial to be more effective in preventing and healing pressure sores than a conventional large-celled ripple bed.

Body moulding mattresses. The alternating pressure mattress works by the periodic relief of pressure which allows the skin to recover. The other approach is to distribute the weight of the body more evenly in order to relieve the circulation in the skin over the bony prominences.

In a patient on an ordinary hospital mattress the interface pressure on the skin over the sacrum is 35−42 mmHg. This is above the normal capillary pressure of the skin which is about 25−30 mmHg. Body moulding mattresses can reduce pressure over the sacrum to between 20−25 mmHg but they have less effect on the heels.

Measuring pressure. The interface pressure between the patient and the bed can be measured by the Talley pressure evaluator. This consists of an inflatable sensor pad connected to a battery operated electric manometer. The sensor pad is inflated by a bulb like that used in a sphygmomanometer.

The sensor is placed under the patient and inflated with air. The air is then released gradually as when taking the blood pressure. As the pressure falls the wires in the sensor complete an electric circuit and a red light glows on the instrument. The pressure at which this first happens is the interface pressure under the patient. It is important to switch off the battery after use.

Foam mattresses. The simplest mattress which will mould itself to the body is one made of soft plastic foam, though it may be enclosed in a frame of tougher plastic to prevent disintegration. The moulding properties of such mattresses are improved if the foam is cut into sections with grooves between them which reduces shearing strain. This is the principle of the Talley Polyfloat mattress. The Astec Clinifloat (Fig. 44) comes in three sections. The middle one can be removed for toileting. The sections are normally enclosed in plastic envelopes but when ventilation is particularly important the uncovered sections may be covered by a special 'microclimate' sheet which is impervious to water but permeable to water vapour. This allows moisture to penetrate the mattress. An electric aerator is used to introduce air into the foam and encourage evaporation.

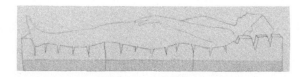

Fig. 44 Clinifloat mattress section

The Courtaulds Vaperm mattress incorporates many of these properties but is designed as a general purpose replacement for the traditional hospital mattress. It is made of foam of several densities. The pressure removing grooves are inside the mattress under a layer of soft foam. It has a special waterproof but moisture permeable cover. It works best on beds with a rigid wire mesh base. Unfortunately most Kings Fund beds have solid bases.

A principle with all these mattresses is that any sheet which covers them must be loose and not tucked in tightly.

The weakness of some of these mattresses at present is the durability of the material. Experience suggests that they may not have a very long life.

Foam and water mattresses. Some mattresses combine the properties of the foam mattress and the water bed.

The Dyson mattress is particularly good. It has two layers. The base is made of high density foam containing in a hollowed out central section three PVC cells which are filled with water. On top of this is placed a mattress of soft foam cut into grooves with ridged sections. This arrangement prevents shearing strain when the patient is sitting up and allows free circulation of air. The foam lying over the water cells conforms exceptionally well to the shape of the patient's body. The whole mattress is covered by flexible material which is waterproof but vapour permeable (Fig. 45 a and b).

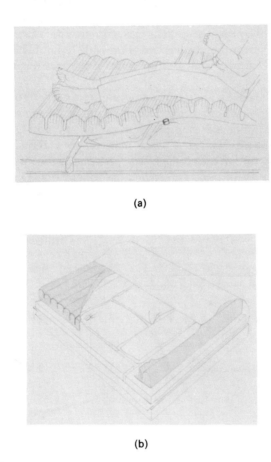

(a)

(b)

Fig. 45 Dyson mattress
    (a) Side view
    (b) Cut-through section

Pressure measurements show results comparable to those obtained with water beds and the facilities for ventilation prevent maceration of the skin. The mattress is comfortable, light and relatively inexpensive. It is acceptable to patients and staff. It does not interfere with rehabilitation because the patient can get in and out of bed in the normal way. There are no electrical or mechanical parts to go wrong. The worst that could happen is a leak in a water bag. This mattress is probably the most promising development in pressure sore prevention for many years.

Water bed. The water bed is simply a mattress shaped bag filled with water. It rests in a metal or plastic tank. The bag should be loosely filled so that the patient can sink into the water but not so deeply that he touches the bottom of the tank. It should be possible to remove the stopper and spill no water if the mattress is correctly filled.

If a person lies on a water bed his weight is evenly distributed and the pressure over bony prominences is reduced. The pressure on the heels and sacrum for example is about $20-25$ mmHg compared with $35-40$ mmHg on a foam mattress or a Ripple bed and 200 mmHg on an operating table. The pressure of blood in the capillaries is 27 mmHg. Thus when the patient is lying on a water bed the blood supply to his skin, even at points of pressure, is still maintained (Fig. 46).

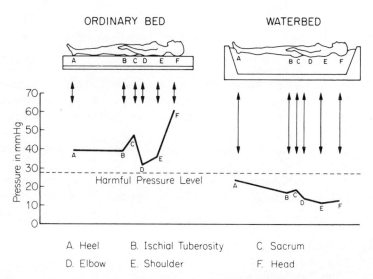

Fig. 46 The water bed distributes the pressure so that a harmful level is avoided

Because the patient would lose heat to the water it has to be warmed electrically. The water should not be too hot, or the patient will sweat and the skin become macerated. If it becomes too cold, through failure of the heating, he may develop hypothermia. For most patients about 30 °C is the best temperature for the water.

The patient is nursed on one sheet and no underblanket is used. A great advantage is that two-hourly turning is unnecessary.

Unfortunately the present types of water beds have many disadvantages. They are extremely heavy and very expensive. The electrical arrangements are not always reliable and if the thermostat is faulty the water may become too hot or too cold. They have to be filled and emptied with a hose and are impossible to move when full. The mattress envelope is liable to puncture and a spare must always be kept on hand. Water beds are only effective when the patient is lying down. It is difficult to use a bed pan or to give an enema. A chemical must be added to the water every few months to prevent the growth of algae. Water beds are bulky to store when not in use.

The best flotation is provided by the sophisticated but very heavy Beaufort water bed whose tank is 15 in deep. The problems of nursing a patient in this environment require special staff training. The Western Medical water bed has a shallower tank and though providing less than perfect flotation is not as heavy and looks more like a conventional bed. It is easier to manage and perhaps more generally acceptable.

Most patients find a water bed acceptable but a few complain of sea sickness and contractures may be likely to develop. The most serious disadvantage, however, is the difficulty of moving the patient in and out of the bed. Water beds should always be used with a gantry hoist and no attempt should be made to lift the patient without this aid (see p. 153). Because it is so difficult to get in and out of the bed, a water bed is unsuitable for patients who are likely to be rehabilitated. It is unsuitable also as a preventative treatment for patients at risk for pressure sores. Its main value is in the treatment of dying patients with pressure sores.

Because water beds are so heavy an attempt has been made to create lighter water mattresses which can be used on an ordinary bed. These are popular in honeymoon hotels but have no place in geriatric medicine.

Net bed

A new concept in pressure sore nursing is the Mecanaids net bed, invented by Mr J. R. Gibbs. The patient is nursed in a hammock suspended from rollers held in a frame which slots into a Kings Fund bed. The hammock can be lowered on to the underlying bed or the patient can be turned by one nurse operating two handles (Fig. 47).

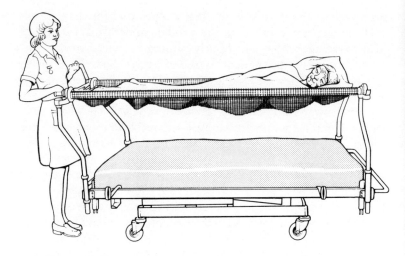

Fig. 47 Net bed. One nurse can turn a patient easily. Pressures under the patient are as low as in a water bed

By lowering the net and removing one roller the patient is enabled to step out of the bed when required.

Pressures under a patient in a net bed are as low as those found in a water bed and sores heal equally well. There are, however, limitations. Because of the height at which the patient is nursed the net bed is unsuitable for the confused, restless patient and for those who have not had time to adjust to life in hospital. For this reason it is not suitable for pressure sore prevention in patients newly admitted to an acute ward for elderly people, where the risk of pressure sores is greatest. Its value lies in treating established pressure sores in co-operative patients with a prospect of rehabilitation.

Low air loss bed

Probably the ultimate and among the most expensive system for the prevention and treatment of pressure sores is the Mediscus low air loss bed (Fig. 48). In essence it is a bed made of 21 air sacs connected to a blower. The sacs are made of permeable material which allows air to escape and ventilate the skin. They thus require continuous inflation from the blower. The pressure in the different sections of the bed can be adjusted according to the patient's weight.

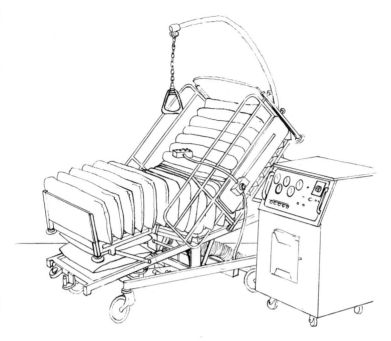

Fig. 48 Mediscus low air loss bed

The air temperature also can be controlled. The patient is assisted in and out across the end of the bed, rather than the side.

The system provides optimal pressure relief and ventilation and is very effective in treating pressure sores but it too has its disadvantages. It is extremely expensive, over £6,000. With its blower and power unit and controls it takes up as much space in the ward as two ordinary beds. As with all complicated machinery breakdowns occur and, unless it is in working order, a very expensive piece of equipment lies useless. A smaller version, the Mediscus Minor, is available. It works on the same principles but the mattress is designed to go on an ordinary domestic or hospital bed. The price is still measured in thousands of pounds, however.

The Clinitron bed

Even more sophisticated (and more expensive) is the Clinitron bed (Support Systems International). The patient lies on a porous sheet which separates him from a tank of glass microspheres no bigger than grains of sand. When warm compressed air is blown through the spheres from the bottom they become 'fluidised' and acquire the properties of a water bed so that the patient sinks into them (Fig. 49a, b and c). The bed may be fluidised continuously or intermittently. The porous sheet allows sweat, urine and secretions to pass into the spheres. Water evaporates and any residual solids fall to the bottom of the tank whence they can be removed. Cleaning takes fifteen minutes a week.

The bed provides excellent flotation and first class ventilation. Apart from its cost its disadvantages are those of the water bed. It is extremely heavy and it is difficult for the patient to get in and out. In some models the heat exchanger, which is needed to keep compressed air at a comfortable temperature, has to be plumbed in.

Which bed?

With such a wealth of technology it is not easy to identify a best buy. The Clinitron is probably the ultimate, but so costly that it can only be had on hire. The low air loss bed is the most practical for the patient with a deep sore and some hope of survival. Every unit needs at least one, despite the cost. Of the ripple beds the Pegasus and the Astec are probably the best but are vulnerable to the main hazard of all ripple beds, human error and poor maintenance. The water bed may be best for the patient who is dying but should be used in conjunction with a hoist, a big disadvantage for a very ill patient. The net bed is fairly expensive but an occasional patient is comfortable on nothing else. The Dyson mattress which combines at low cost the advantages of a foam mattress and a water bed is probably the best buy for the patient at high risk for sores. Every ward should have at least one.

Treatment of established pressure sores

The occurrence of a superficial sore is a sign to step up the preventive measures already described. It is not serious in itself and will soon heal. A deep sore, on the other hand, is a disaster that threatens the patient's life.

Local treatment. Erythema alone requires only continued application of preventive measures. Blisters normally burst under natural pressures. Superficial sores respond well to povidone iodine in a dry powder spray, Disadine DP. If an occlusive dressing is required Op-Site applied direct to the skin protects it and allows ventilation. It is helpful also to sit the patient on a nursing fleece.

A urine rash will respond to improved ventilation and to the

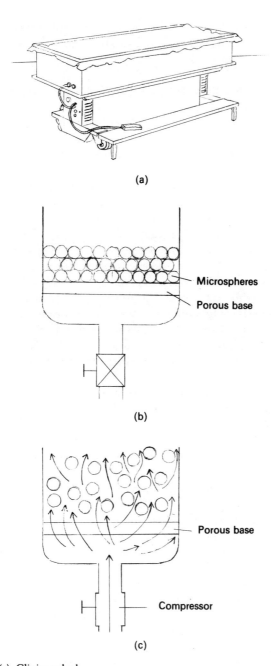

Fig. 49 (a) Clinitron bed
(b) Clinitron bed at rest – compacted
(c) Clinitron bed fluidised

application of benzalkonium, Drapolene. Sometimes there is fungal infection as well and a fungicidal ointment such as clotrimazole, Canesten, will help to clear it up.

Deep sores. The first problem with a deep sore is the removal of the slough. It can be cut away with sterile scissors but this is probably not necessary. Nature will provide the enzymes to separate the slough in one or two weeks. Enzyme preparations such as Varidase have been claimed to accelerate the separation of the slough but there is little evidence to support this.

Deep sores should not be packed. Dr Bliss points out that packing keeps the sore open, prevents discharge, interferes with the growth of granulation tissue and increases ischaemia.

There is no need to maintain patency in these large freely draining cavities. The sooner they are allowed to close by contraction the better. They do not need to be encouraged to granulate from the bottom, as they do this naturally.

A deep sore should be left completely empty, without even a swab placed in the cavity to level it up. It should be dressed simply with sheets of gauze and strapping bridged across the mouth of the wound to absorb the discharge. Occlusive dressings are difficult to secure in the sacral region, but tubular elasticated net bandage is very useful.

Incontinent patients with deep pressure sores are usually catheterised though there is no very good evidence to support the need for this practice.

It is unnecessary to use any antiseptics or antibiotics to sterilise the wound. Necrotic material always contains numerous organisms. These will do no harm and will help to break down the slough. Local antiseptics can impede this process by damaging surrounding granulation tissue. Systemic antibiotics should not be used unless there is evidence of septicaemia.

To clean the wound nothing more is required than irrigation with normal saline once or twice daily. Eusol should be avoided. It may be painful and can impair wound healing.

If any local application is used it should be a substance which increases secretion and discharge from the wound. In the past honey was used for this purpose. Its modern alternative is dextranomer (Debrisan). Not all large pressure sores will heal completely. Often the patient will die. But if he seems likely to survive it is worth consulting a plastic surgeon.

Heel sores. No local application is of proven value. A nonadherent dry dressing may be all that is needed. A deep sore will take several months to heal.

A most important point about heel sores is that they should not be allowed to prevent the patient from walking. Heel sores are usually on the back of the heel and not on the sole where weight is taken when the patient walks.

General measures. The most important general measure is to treat the patient energetically for the illness which led to his acquiring a pressure sore. In addition a high protein diet can be given to replace the protein lost in the discharge from the ulcer. Vitamin C may also be given in large doses (1.0 g per day). This has been shown to reduce the incidence of pressure sores after surgical operations. Most patients with pressure sores are also anaemic. Haematinics are rarely effective but a blood transfusion is often useful. Finally zinc sulphate given by mouth in a dose of 220 mg tds may be helpful. Unless the patient is dying most pressure sores will heal eventually but sometimes treatment by a surgeon is needed before they will do so.

Monitoring treatment. The best way to monitor the progress of a pressure sore is to photograph it regularly with a polaroid camera. This produces a picture which can immediately be filed in the notes. It is important to include a ruler or tape measure in the picture to give it scale.

For further reading:

BARBENEL, J. C., FORBES, C. D. & LOWE, G. D. O. 1983. *Pressure Sores.* London: Macmillan.

See also:

Care, Science and Practice. The journal of Society for Tissue Viability. 1981. Vol. 1. Odstock Hospital, Salisbury.

17
Continence and Bladder Problems

Incontinence in hospital is a problem for up to 1 in 3 of patients in geriatric wards, and about 1 in 8 in general wards. In the community some degree of incontinence has been reported by 11 per cent of elderly women and 7 per cent of men. Incontinence causes misery and humiliation to the patient, great burdens to those who care for him and a heavy cost to the National Health Service.

Incontinence is a symptom, not a diagnosis. It has many causes. To understand these it is helpful to consider first the workings of the normal bladder.

The normal bladder

The normal bladder in an old person has a capacity of 250–500 ml. It fills at the rate of 1–2 ml per minute or 60–120 ml per hour, depending on how much is drunk. Thus a small bladder in a person who is drinking well may be almost full after two hours. As it fills the muscular wall of the bladder, the detrusor, stretches. There is no increase in pressure but the increased muscle tension eventually communicates itself to consciousness as a desire to pass water. A normal person of any age can restrain his bladder emptying until a convenient moment. This process is known as inhibition. In younger people the desire to void may reach consciousness when the bladder is only half full, but in normal old people awareness of this need may not be felt until the bladder is almost full to capacity.

Micturition

During the period of inhibition the sphincters in the urethra itself and in the muscles of the pelvic floor ensure that the pressure in the urethra is greater than the pressure within the bladder. And so continence is preserved. When inhibition is lifted the sphincters relax and urethral pressure falls. Meanwhile the detrusor contracts and raises the pressure within the bladder. As soon as pressure within the bladder exceeds that in the urethra urine is passed. The rate at which urine is passed is reduced in older people. If there is any obstruction to the urinary outflow or weakness of the detrusor it will be reduced still further.

The unstable bladder

Some elderly people, especially those with a tendency to incontinence, have what is called an unstable bladder. Contractions of the detrusor, giving rise to increase in pressure, may occur when there is only a small volume of urine in the bladder. These contractions may be sufficient to overcome the normal resistance of the sphincters so that leakage occurs. Unstable bladders are commonly of small capacity and residual urine may exceed 100 ml. Detrusor contractions may occur spontaneously as the bladder fills or they may be provoked by coughing and straining. Bladder instability is common in children with enuresis and may persist throughout life. In the elderly it is often associated with neurological impairment, for example stroke, Parkinsonism or dementia.

A person who has to empty his bladder as soon as he is aware of the need to do so is said to suffer from urgency and this is the main symptom of the unstable bladder. Because of the small capacity and residual urine only a little additional urine is needed to trigger another bladder contraction. So urgency is often associated with frequency and the patient fails either to fill or empty his bladder completely.

Urge incontinence

A patient with urgency and frequency due to an unstable bladder is at risk of becoming incontinent. If this occurs it is known as urge incontinence. This is the commonest type of bladder problem in old age.

Urge incontinence is not, however, an all or none affair. It depends on many factors, personal and environmental.

Mobility

Many people with bladder instability remain continent provided they can reach the lavatory and manage their clothing within about two minutes of the desire to void. This is why it is advocated that lavatories should be situated within 10 m (33 ft) of patient areas in wards for the elderly. Incontinence is likely if mobility is impaired for any reason, for example acute illness, depression, inertia or pain.

Environment

Continence may be lost if, as a result of transfer to hospital or an old people's home, a patient finds himself in an unfamiliar environment. Anyone whose custom has been to get out of bed in the night to pass urine will be incontinent if he is placed in a high hospital bed and cannot get out of it. The situation is compounded if he is imprisoned with cot sides.

In the daytime incontinence will occur if the lavatory is too far away, if the patient does not know or cannot remember where it is, if there is no one available to help him walk there, or if he has to wait in a queue when he arrives.

Psychological

The bladder is a sensitive emotional barometer. Anyone who has taken an examination or been for an interview knows that anxiety impairs the power to inhibit the bladder and provokes frequency. In the elderly loneliness, boredom and family tension can all have similar effects.

Drugs

Drugs can predispose to incontinence. Diuretics given to patients with impaired mobility may provoke incontinence. Tranquillisers and sleeping tablets which reduce the patient's awareness of his bladder and perhaps his mobility are also well known precipitants of incontinence.

Local factors

Acute urinary infections increase the sensitivity of the stretch receptors in the bladder wall and may provoke incontinence.

Chronic urinary infections, on the other hand, are commonly seen in patients who are already habitually incontinent. They are often associated with the presence of residual urine. Treatment of the infection does not usually sterilise the urine for long and has no effect on the incontinence. Chronic urinary infections are therefore regarded as an accompaniment rather than a cause of incontinence.

Senile vaginitis is another cause of incontinence. Lack of oestrogen leads not only to atrophy of the vagina but also to shrinkage of the cells of the urethra. Urethral closure is less secure and urethral resistance is more easily overcome by an unstable bladder contraction.

Distortion of the bladder from without, particularly at its neck, is an important factor provoking incontinence. Prostatic hypertrophy is itself a cause of bladder instability but it may also cause accumulation of residual urine and thus frequency. Bladder capacity may be reduced by pressure from without by pelvic tumours, but the common cause in the elderly is constipation with or without faecal impaction.

Overflow incontinence

Overflow incontinence is associated with retention of urine. It is sometimes known as retention with overflow. Incontinence occurs when the pressure within the bladder exceeds the urethral resistance, but this may not happen until there is a large volume of urine. Because the bladder wall is overstretched effective detrusor contraction does not occur and the urine leaks only in small quantities.

The patient often complains of frequency and may have a sense of incomplete emptying. He may have to strain to pass urine at all. The principal physical finding is a great enlargement of the bladder which can be seen and felt through the abdominal wall.

The usual cause of overflow incontinence in men is enlargement of the prostate or occasionally urethral stricture. In women there may be fibrosis of the bladder neck. In both sexes painless enlargement of the bladder may accompany neurological illness such as stroke, Parkinsonism or diabetic neuropathy. One of the most important causes is faecal impaction.

Stress incontinence

Stress incontinence is the name given to the leakage of urine which occurs at moments of increased intra-abdominal pressure. The patient, almost always a woman, loses a small amount of urine when she laughs, sneezes, coughs or strains. The increased intra-abdominal pressure is transmitted passively to the bladder and is sufficient, for a moment, to overcome the urethral resistance, but there is no contraction of the detrusor. Stress incontinence is sometimes known as incontinence due to sphincter weakness or sphincter incompetence. Stress incontinence begins in middle life or earlier. It is often the result of damage to the pelvic floor in childbirth.

Stress incontinence due to sphincter incompetence alone is unusual in the elderly. What is more common is stress-induced detrusor contraction in a patient with an unstable bladder. The stress does not produce immediate passive leakage of a little urine. Rather, after a moment's delay, there is an active contraction of the detrusor with a full emptying of the bladder and the passage of copious urine. This is what happens when an old lady floods the floor on rising from her chair, a not uncommon situation.

Medical investigation

The cause of the incontinence will always be sought. Rectal examination may reveal constipation or faecal impaction. It also enables the prostate to be considered in men and the pelvic organs in women. The urine will be tested for sugar and for evidence of infection. This may be followed by an intravenous urogram or ultrasound examination to show the function of the kidneys and bladder and to estimate the amount of residual urine. If the hospital has a urodynamic service, pressure and volume changes in the bladder may be studied directly. Occasionally cystoscopy will be indicated.

Medical treatment of incontinence

Unconscious patients will be incontinent and need catheterisation. So will those whose incontinence is due to retention with overflow. Incontinence due to acute illness, including urinary infections, will respond to the appropriate treatment.

Where urge incontinence persists a number of drugs will be tried, though none with any great hope of success. The main group of drugs used for incontinence all have an atropine-like action. This makes the bladder less irritable and reduces urgency and frequency. Commonly used drugs in this group include oxybutanin (Cystrin) flavoxate (Urispas), emepronium bromide (Cetiprin) and imipramine (Tofranil). All these drugs cause some drying of the mouth and a tendency to constipation. They may cause dilatation of the pupil and increase the pressure within the eye. For this reason they are not used for patients with glaucoma. Emepronium bromide has a bitter taste and can cause ulceration of the mouth and of the oesophagus. It should always be given with plenty of water so that it is swallowed quickly and does not linger in the mouth or gullet. All these drugs should be given at a time when incontinence is most likely. This is usually at night. Another substance which helps women with incontinence is the sex hormone, oestrogen. This is of value when the incontinence is associated with atrophic vaginitis. By increasing the quality of the cells lining the bladder outlet oestrogen improves the closure of the urethra.

Observation

Drugs given for incontinence are often unsuccessful and good nurse management is the mainstay of treatment. This begins with accurate observation. It is important to try to determine the pattern of the patient's incontinence. Is he wet at night only or by day and night, and if so at what time? Or does he merely have the occasional accident? Does he have control of his bladder under conditions of self-care, or only when the nurse takes the initiative, what Dr John Agate calls 'nurse controlled continence'? Details should be recorded in the nursing notes.

In difficult cases it is helpful to use the chart devised by Professor J. C. Brocklehurst (Fig. 50). The nurse attends the patient every two hours, offers him toilet facilities and records whether he is wet or dry. This activity, although expensive in nurse time, is therapeutic in itself and may enable the patient to regain control of his bladder.

Other charts are available for patients able to keep their own records. These are increasingly used in incontinence clinics.

Promotion of continence

It is helpful to think less of incontinence as a disease to be treated and more of continence as a state which can be actively promoted. The essential principle is to create a secure, relaxed environment where the patient can feel accepted and at ease. Occupation is important also. A bored patient is more likely to be wet. It is remarkable how little incontinence occurs on an outing.

The patient should be dressed in his own clothes. If he is in a day room with a choice of interesting things to do he is much more likely to control his bladder. He must be encouraged to go to the lavatory as often as necessary. Three-hourly toilet rounds suit most people but the nurse must explain, particularly to the newly arrived patient, where the lavatories are and how to get help at other times. She must also understand that the older patient's call for help with toilet is urgent and cannot be deferred.

No patient should use a bed pan if he can get to a commode and he should not use a commode, except perhaps at night, if he can get to the lavatory. Sometimes admission to hospital breaks the patient's habit of bladder control and regular visits to the toilet may help to restore this. The nurse who spends time escorting the patient to the lavatory is making the most important contribution to his rehabilitation. She is also helping him regain his self-respect, for few things are more humiliating than dependence on others in toilet matters. Once he gets to the lavatory he needs privacy and time.

INCONTINENCE CHART

SURNAME	FIRST NAMES	UNIT NO.

WARD ....

Date											
Time	Commode or Bed Pan Given by	Urine Faeces or Dry	Commode or Bed Pan Given by	Urine Faeces or Dry	Commode or Bed Pan Given by	Urine Faeces or Dry	Commode or Bed Pan Given by	Urine Faeces or Dry	Commode or Bed Pan Given by	Urine Faeces or Dry	Commode or Bed Pan Given by	Urine Faeces or Dry
8												
10												
12												
14												
16												
18												
20												
22												
24												
2												
4												
6												

Fluid control

The patient who is incontinent should not be deprived of fluid as this may lead to dehydration and to the passage of concentrated urine which is itself irritating to the bladder. It is, however, reasonable not to give large quantities of fluid in the evening, a point which many old people discover for themselves.

The difficult patient

In a small but trying minority of patients the incontinence is likely to be associated with a disorder of behaviour. The patient, although taken regularly to the toilet, does nothing while he is there, but wets himself as soon as he returns. To deal with this situation needs all the nurse's skill and tolerance. Scolding and punishment have no place. Kindness and refusal to take offence are far more effective. When the patient feels secure he will regain control.

For further reading:

JORDAN, J. A. & STANTON, S. K. (Eds). 1981. *The Incontinent Woman.* Royal College of Obstetricians and Gynaecologists.
MANDELSTAM, D. 1977. *Incontinence: A Guide to the Understanding and Management of a Common Complaint.* London: Heinemann.

18
Management of Incontinence

Even the best nursing team is bound to meet patients whose incontinence is not controlled by habit retraining. For them special techniques and equipment are needed. Disposable polythene gloves, paper tissues and wipes have made the nurse's tasks much easier.

Underpads

Disposable incontinence underpads are used extensively. In the community they are invaluable. In hospital, where staff should be available to promote continence day and night, fewer should be needed.

The standard size is 60 cm × 40 cm but there are larger and smaller pads available. Incontinence underpads consist of layers of absorbent material sandwiched between a cover of one way fabric and a waterproof backing. In most types the constituents are bonded along the long side only and it is important that they are placed across the bed and not lengthwise. If this is not done the urine is squeezed out of the open ends by the patient's weight and neither he nor the bed is protected. Some recent types are bonded on all four sides and can be used in any position. Another advance is to incorporate a deodorant in the pad.

If the underpad is to work efficiently the patient must sit on it without any clothes intervening. Women should wear a short nightdress or a split back gown, men a pyjama jacket. For this reason, although widely used, the pads are unsuitable for patients in chairs. Although they protect the chair well enough they do nothing for the patient who must sit with no clothing below the waist except perhaps a blanket. This is an unacceptable affront to anyone's self-respect.

There are many varieties of underpad. The best and most expensive will absorb a litre of urine. Cheaper pads absorb about 300 ml. They are suitable only for the patient who is occasionally incontinent and whose leakage is small. The cheaper pads tend to move around the bed and crease under the patient. Once the surface breaks the pad readily disintegrates and fragments of wadding adhere to the patient's skin. All underpads are difficult to place under the patient and to remove from the bed while he is lying in it. It is usually necessary to roll the patient first on to one side and then on to the other as when changing a draw sheet. The skin should be washed and dried when the pad is changed.

All incontinence pads are designed to be used one at a time. As each pad has a waterproof backing there is no advantage in putting one on top of another.

Kylie absorbent bed sheet

The Kylie absorbent bed sheet is a draw sheet 96 cm × 98 cm. It consists of a layer of water repellent brushed nylon quilted to an absorbent layer of needled rayon. A Kylie pad can absorb up to 2.5 l of urine, more than any patient is likely to pass in 24 hours and the surface will remain dry. The Kylie has side flaps of polyester cotton to tuck under the mattress and hold it in place. Unlike a disposable incontinent underpad it does not have built in waterproof backing and must be used in conjunction with a waterproof sheet to protect the bed (Fig. 51).

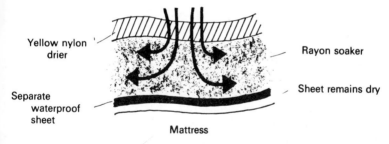

Yellow nylon drier

Rayon soaker

Separate waterproof sheet

Sheet remains dry

Mattress

Fig. 51 Kylie absorbent bed sheet structure

Kylies are very comfortable and popular with patients. Because they need changing less often they ease the work of the nurse.

The initial cost of Kylies has limited their use but they have a long life and compared with the expense of disposables they can be cost effective.

They require a special washing programme which not all hospital laundries are at present organised to provide.

Kylies are of particular value for patients at home, provided the household possesses a washing machine and a tumble dryer. The Kylies should be washed with detergent, not soap. They should not be boiled but can be disinfected with bleach. Fabric softeners impair the absorbency of the material and should be avoided. Kylies should not be ironed.

Incontinence pants and pads

Incontinence pants provide valuable reassurance to patients who are liable to have the occasional accident. They are designed to hold an absorbent pad between the legs as close as possible to the opening of the urethra. Pads hold up to 450 ml of urine. If the patient is regularly incontinent they must be changed whenever they are wet. The pads may be made with or without their own waterproof plastic backing. The modern trend is towards a T-shaped pad which gives greater comfort and protection. In one system the material is provided in a roll from which the user cuts as much as is necessary to meet his needs.

An expensive version is the Gelulose incontinence pad. This is like an ordinary sanitary towel but the absorbent material consists of powdered cellulose which on contact with urine forms an odourless gel. These pads will hold up to 150 ml of urine, but they may cause some stickiness of the vulva.

Pants

Incontinence pants are of three types.

Waterproof pants. There is the traditional plastic incontinence pants used with disposable interliners. These do not allow the skin to breathe. They do not separate the patient from his urine. They are liable to cause a rash. Increasingly they are being superseded by more sophisticated models.

Marsupial pants. A great advance was the invention of the marsupial pant by Dr F. L. Willington. Marsupial pants hold the absorbent pad in a waterproof pouch on the outside of the garment (Fig. 52). The pant is made of one-way water repellant fabric which remains dry while allowing the urine to pass through into a disposable double folded pad. There is no need to remove the pants when the pad is changed becuase the pouch is on the outside. But some skill is needed to ensure that the pad is properly positioned.

To be effective the pants must fit tightly like swimming trunks. They come in a number of sizes determined by the patient's hip

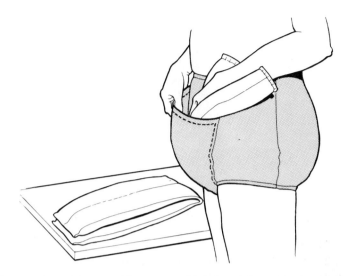

Fig. 52 Marsupial pants with waterproof pouch and disposable absorbent pad

measurement and must be fitted accurately. Moreover, time must be spent teaching the patient how to use the pants. His family also must feel that they understand them. Marsupial pants are of limited value at night because the urine tends to pool at the back of the pad. This is less likely to be a problem, however, if the pad is pushed as far back as possible. To allow for washing, one patient needs three pairs of pants. Not all patients find marsupial pants acceptable. Some feel they are too bulky. The original marsupial pants were marketed as Kanga pants but there are now a number of versions on the market, including special models with fly openings for men.

Elastic stretch pants. The third type of pants are elastic stretch pants. They provide no protection on their own but hold in place a pad with its own waterproof backing. There are many brands on the market. Their main advantage is their lightness. The elastic material is so versatile that size is seldom critical. They are perhaps more popular with those who manage their own incontinence than for patients in hospital (Fig. 53).

Disposable Pants. There are also disposable pants. Some are designed to hold a separate pad in place, for example the Mölnlycke Snibb, an elegant bikini with tie fastening.

Others include an integral pad, for example Vernon Carus Protecta pants, or the adult diapers marketed as Incontinettes by Ancilla or as Cumfies by Vernon Carus.

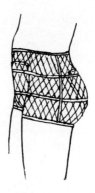

Fig. 53 Elastic stretch pant used with waterproof backed pad

They are fastened with adhesive strips and are generally more convenient than the pull on pants which usually have to be cut off with scissors when they are wet.

The most sophisticated disposable pant is the Ancilla Tender, a drop front model in which the absorbent material is covered by a one way fabric and the legs are elasticated for a closer fit.

Which pants?

No one type of incontinence pant or liner can suit everybody. An attempt should be made to find what is most acceptable to the individual patient. Choice in hospital may be restricted by unimaginative purchasing policies.

Patients with only a moderate loss of urine do not need bulky pads of high absorbency. For them the stylish Kanga Lady pants whose pads hold only 200 ml are likely to be very acceptable.

Those who need larger pads can choose between standard marsupial pants and a waterproof backed pad, for example Smith and Nephew's Dandeliners or Mölnlycke's T pads. On the whole marsupial pads require some dexterity and are probably best suited to dependent patients for whom the nurse changes the pad. Many patients find them rather bulky. A waterproof-backed pad worn under close-fitting pants is often preferred by patients who change their own pads. Gelulose pads are liked by a few patients but are not available on NHS prescription.

Drop front pants can be changed in the sitting position and are often the best for the patient in a wheelchair. Side opening pants can be put on while the patient lies in bed. Both types are available in marsupial or conventional form.

Disposable pants save laundry and provide good protection. But some nurses feel that they are too like a baby's nappy and infantilise the patient.

Disposal

The disposal of incontinence pads is always a problem. They cannot be put down the lavatory. Most Local Authorities supply users with waterproof bags which are collected periodically for incineration.

Personal urinals

The urine bottle for men has not changed in many years except that it is now made of plastic rather than glass or metal. But it has recently become possible to improve it with a lid or non-spill adaptor to prevent leakage (Fig. 54a).

For women there are two small personal urinals which can be very

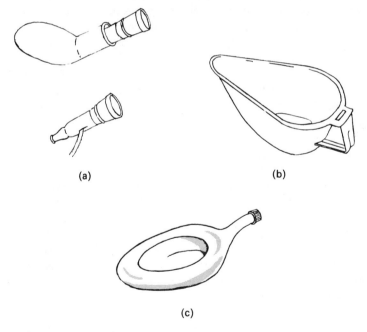

(a)　　　　　　　　　　(b)

(c)

Fig. 54 Personal Urinals
     (a) Non-spill adaptor for male urinal
     (b) St. Peter's boat
     (c) Suba-Seal urinal

useful. The St. Peter's boat can be positioned between the legs and used while standing. It can also be used in the sitting position at the edge of the bed or at the front of a chair (Fig. 54b).

The Suba-Seal urinal is a small shallow plastic bedpan with a capped hollow handle through which it is emptied. It can be slipped under the buttocks without raising the hips and some women find it particularly useful at night (Fig. 54c).

Male incontinence aids

Some incontinence pants and pads are specifically designed for men. The Kanga Male marsupial pant has a fly opening but it requires considerable dexterity to use it effectively. The Lic drop shield and the Mölnlycke maxi pocket pad are small bags containing absorbent material. They are placed over the penis and held in position by close fitting pants.

Some men find a condom urinal more acceptable. There are many varieties on the market. The Bard Urosheath and the Coloplast Convene are perhaps two of the best. Successful use of these aids depends on the intelligent co-operation of the patient. Unfortunately this is just what is lacking in many old men whose incontinence is associated with mental impairment and immobility. A good use for a condom urinal is to help the patient who is temporarily incontinent after prostatic surgery.

A very small or retracted penis may make any form of condom drainage impossible.

Catheterisation

Catheterisation over a long period leads to contraction of the bladder and negates efforts to restore bladder control. Catheters passed for the temporary relief of incontinence in very ill patients should be withdrawn as soon as possible so that bladder rehabilitation can begin.

Nevertheless there is a place in certain patients for long term catheterisation. It is a treatment of last resort but is of undoubted value when all other measures have failed. Sometimes long-term catheterisation enables people to live at home when this would not otherwise be possible.

A Foley self-retaining catheter is used. The catheter should not be too large. Sizes 14, 16 or 18 FG are usually best. A 5 or 10 ml balloon is preferable to a larger one. The smaller balloon is less likely to irritate the bladder and cause painful spasm or leakage. An important advance has been the introduction of the short catheter for women.

This is 21 cm long, about half the length of a conventional male catheter.

Catheter bags

The catheter drains into a bag. This may be strapped to the thigh, above or below the knee, suspended from a waistband in a sporran or, increasingly often, inserted into a pouch in a special undergarment. Women normally prefer a bag above the knee and men a bag below. The best bags are backed with a layer of non-woven fabric. This makes for greater comfort and reduces skin irritation. Leg bags have a capacity of between 250 and 500 ml. The most sophisticated ones are partitioned to prevent urine slopping about. Bags normally need emptying three or four times a day. The problem which has not yet been entirely solved is the provision of an outlet tap which can be manipulated by one hand without soiling the fingers. Bags fastened to the legs with plastic straps may be uncomfortable and foam and velcro bands are preferred by most patients. Two bands are always necessary at the top and bottom of the bag. It is important that the bag should be properly supported at all times. It must not hang down, pulling on the catheter. At night the bag is probably best left lying free in the bed, though being of small volume it may need emptying. Some people prefer to exchange the small day bag for a night bag of larger volume which normally stands by the bed on a frame. A useful innovation is the night bag which can be connected via a length of plastic tubing to the outlet tap of the day bag.

Catheter problems

Latex catheters need changing after a week. They block easily because the wall is thick and the lumen relatively small. Plastic catheters have a larger lumen, a thinner wall and last longer. The more expensive all silicone catheters have the largest lumen in relation to their size and are the least likely to irritate the urethra and bladder. They are also less likely to become encrusted with precipitates and may last for a month or longer before needing to be changed. Encrustation seems to be an individual matter and some patients are more prone to it than others. All catheters work better if the patient is taking plenty to drink and passing a dilute urine.

Some elderly patients eventually develop leakage around the catheter, a common reason being catheter blockage. It is best to change the catheter when this occurs. If this fails the temptation is to try a larger catheter but in fact a smaller one, and sometimes a smaller balloon, is more likely to be effective.

Painful spasm around the catheter can be treated with flavoxate. If the balloon does not collapse when the catheter has to be withdrawn it can usually be deflated by introducing a needle into the side tube just above the valve. If this does not work expert help is needed and the urologist should be consulted. It is particularly important not to cut the catheter across. If this is done the operator loses control of the situation and the subsequent removal of the catheter is made more difficult.

All patients on long-term catheterisation have a chronic urinary infection, but for the most part this does them no harm. Regular bladder washouts and instillations of noxythiolin were in vogue a few years ago but have largely been abandoned. All forms of long-term antibiotic or antiseptic treatment are equally ineffective. Sometimes however the patient develops an acute or chronic urinary infection with troublesome symptoms. A short course of a broad spectrum antibiotic will then bring symptomatic relief though it will not sterilise the urine.

Smell

Any smell associated with incontinence can be dispelled by Nilodor. This comes in a bottle with a single drop dispenser. One drop on the patient's underclothes will dispel offensive odours for many hours. It can also be added to the rinsing water when the clothes are washed.

Continence nurse advisers

The field of incontinence equipment has become so complex and changes so often that it is difficult to keep up-to-date. For this reason some nurses have been appointed as continence advisers to counsel patients, assist in their investigation and to evaluate new equipment. There is a lively Association of Continence Advisers (ACA). The Association has produced an excellent directory of aids. The address is the same as the Disabled Living Foundation (p. xi).

For further reading:

ASSOCIATION OF CONTINENCE ADVISORS. 1983. *Association of Continence Advisors Directory of Aids.*

JOHNSON, A. 1984. *Guidelines for the Management of the Catheterised Patient.* Sunderland: Bard Ltd.

MENDELSTAM, D. (Ed). 1980. *Incontinence and Its Management.* Beckenham: Croom Helm.

19
The Bowel and Toilet Facilities

The elderly are much concerned with their bowels and a few introspective individuals appear to think of little else. Today's old people were brought up in an era when much ill health was attributed to constipation. The weekly purgative was a ritual in many families and even today one old person in three maintains the habit.

The normal bowel

When the contents of the intestine enter the large bowel through the ileo–caecal valve they are liquid. When passed as faeces they have become solid. In their journey down the colon much water is absorbed and their bulk is reduced by four-fifths. The rectum is normally empty and the faeces are stored in the sigmoid colon. From time to time the bowel propels faeces into the rectum and when this happens a call to stool is felt. This desire can be inhibited if there is no convenient opportunity for defaecation. If ignored the desire goes away but returns later when more faeces pass into the rectum. By getting the patient to swallow a marker which can be identified when it appears in the faeces it is possible to measure the 'transit time' of food through the body.

The bowel in old age

In the healthy old person a marker reaches the lower bowel in about three days and is passed promptly. The transit time is about the same as in the young. In the infirm old person, however, there is a diminished awareness of the rectum. The call to stool is weak or not felt at all. The passage of faeces through the colon is not necessarily much delayed but the faeces are retained in the rectum and sigmoid for long periods, sometimes increasing the transit time to two or three weeks. In a few cases the rectum and colon may become greatly dilated to accommodate the retained faeces. The condition is then called megacolon.

Constipation

Constipation implies the abnormal retention of faecal matter in the bowel. Whether a patient complains of it depends partly on his expectations. Many people who think they are constipated and take a purgative regularly continue to have regular bowel actions when the purgatives are stopped. Constipation may be due to delayed passage through the colon or the retention of faeces in the lower bowel and rectum. Often both factors are combined.

Delayed passage through the colon may be due to poor diet with too little fluid and too little fibre. Many drugs reduce the activity of the colon. They include codeine, morphine, iron, calcium, atropine and substances related to it, which are used to relieve spasm, Parkinsonism and depression.

Abnormal retention of faeces in the rectum may be due to the diminished awareness already mentioned. Confinement to bed and muscular weakness make the act of defaecation difficult and incomplete. Painful conditions of the rectum and anus may make the patient reluctant to go to the lavatory. The toilet facilities themselves may contribute. Nothing makes it harder for a patient to open his bowels than to have to balance on a bedpan. A warm accessible lavatory is an invitation to a good bowel habit. A cold, distant, outside toilet is the reverse.

Faecal retention

Prolonged constipation leads to the accumulation of a mass of faeces in the rectum. This is called faecal retention. Faecal retention may make the patient restless and confused. It may lead to retention of urine, or to vomiting and abdominal distention. By far the commonest consequence however is faecal overflow. Some faeces come away but the rectum never empties completely. The faeces which leak under these circumstances are fairly soft and have a pungent odour.

Faecal impaction

Less commonly the faeces become hardened into a mass like a cricket ball which acts as a ball valve, liquid faeces mixed with mucus trickling around the obstruction from above. Any of the urinary and intestinal complications of faecal retention may occur and there may be on rare occasions intestinal obstruction. Patients may complain of a bearing down sensation.

Faecal incontinence

Faecal retention and faecal impaction are the commonest causes of faecal incontinence and should be assumed to be present until proved otherwise. There are, however, other causes. In a patient with severe brain damage automatic emptying of the rectum may occur without massive impaction. This is known as automatic or uninhibited neurogenic rectum.

Prolapse of the rectum deprives the patient of an effective anal sphincter and is an occasional cause of intractable faecal incontinence.

Faecal incontinence may also be due to true diarrhoea caused by over-treatment with purgatives. In addition diseases of the bowel, such as gastroenteritis, cancer of the rectum and diverticular disease may all cause diarrhoea and faecal incontinence.

Rectal examination

Most of the causes of faecal incontinence can be identified by rectal examination. In true diarrhoea the rectum is normally empty and the faeces are runny and often pale in colour. In faecal retention the rectum is loaded. Prolapsed rectum is immediately revealed to the eye. Rectal examination is an essential part of the doctor's investigation of the older patient but in cases of faecal incontinence the nurse should be prepared to examine the rectum herself. After a word of explanation she introduces a gloved and lubricated finger into the rectum. There is nothing difficult or dangerous about this procedure. It is immensely informative and readiness to perform it when the patient has faecal incontinence is one of the hallmarks of a nurse well trained in the care of the elderly.

Treatment of faecal retention and impaction

It is useless to give a purgative to a patient with faecal retention. It is likely to cause abdominal pain and will not clear the bowel. It is essential to tackle the problem from below. It is never enough to rely on a single enema. The enemas should be repeated daily (or on alternate days if the patient is very frail), until the bowel can be proved empty by an examining finger. This usually takes a week or longer. In the worse cases it may be necessary to begin with a manual removal.

Disposable phosphate enemas are preferred by most nurses but the citrate micro-enemas (Micralax, Micolett, Relaxit) with a volume of only 5 ml have their enthusiastic advocates. Klyx enemas containing sorbitol and a wetting agent dioctyl in 120 ml of fluid are also satisfactory. If the faecal mass is very hard an oil retention enema can be used to soften it. Fletcher's arachis oil enema (130 ml) in a disposable pack with a long nozzle is very convenient. The patient should be encouraged to retain the oil for at least three hours. It may help to raise the foot of the bed.

In milder cases bisacodyl (Dulcolax) suppositories 10 mg may be used. Beogex suppositories which stimulate the bowel by the release of carbon dioxide and the time honoured glycerine suppositories are more gentle but less effective. Suppositories, though easier to administer than enemas, tend to produce incomplete but prolonged bowel action in frailer patients. For the more robust they are invaluable.

Occasionally when the rectum has been emptied the faecal incontinence persists. This suggests retention of faeces higher up in the colon, a point which can be demonstrated by an X-ray picture of the abdomen. Persistence with enemas for a few more days will usually clear it.

After treatment

After a bout of faecal retention the nurse must pay special attention to the patient's bowels. If she assists the patient with a bowel action she should record the result immediately. It is not enough to enquire if the bowels have acted. The older patient may be forgetful or give a misleading answer.

The patient should be given plenty of time on the lavatory or commode. Every effort should be made to improve his mobility and to ensure that he takes as much fluid and fibre as possible. A laxative is usually given if the patient has been three days without a bowel action. It may be given earlier if requested. The nurse should not be misled by incomplete evacuation. The patient who appears to have had a motion may in fact have passed only a small amount and failed to clear the rectum. For the same reason a negative enema result does not prove that the rectum is empty. Rectal examination is the only reliable guide.

Aperients

Aperient, laxative and purgative all mean the same thing, a substance given to relieve constipation. The most physiological, but not always the most acceptable, are the substances which put fibre into the diet, absorb water and add bulk to the faeces. Two dessertspoonsful of bran, taken with porridge, cornflakes or soup, shorten transit time and increase the weight of the stool. Bran breakfast cereals and bran biscuits are sometimes more acceptable. Other bulk laxatives which work in the same way, but are more obviously medicines include sterculia gum, ispaghula husks, psyllium seeds and synthetic methylcellulose. Fybogel and Regulan contain ispaghula in a form that makes an effervescent drink. However, if not drunk at once, it turns into a less palatable gel.

Saline purgatives like magnesium sulphate (Epsom salts) tend to produce a liquid stool and are better avoided. Lactulose syrup (Duphalac, Gatinar) contains synthetic sugar. It is broken down by the bacteria of the colon into organic acids which work in a rather similar way to a saline purgative. Lactulose is gentle and safe, but it has an extremely sweet taste and is rather expensive. The detergent Dioctyl is useful and safe. It softens the stool without stimulating the bowel.

Of preparations which stimulate the colon directly Senokot, a standardised preparation of senna, is very satisfactory either as a syrup, as granules taken with water or in tablet form. Another liquid preparation is sodium picosulphate (Laxoberal). Bisacodyl (Dulcolax) tablets may be given by mouth in the evening. Next morning, if necessary, a further dose may be given as a suppository. This regime sometimes causes griping but saves many enemas. It has proved valuable in continuing care wards.

A very popular alternative is co-danthromer (Dorbanex) which contains a chemical laxative, danthron, with a softening agent poloxamer. Duclodos, a tablet which combines bisacodyl with docusate (Dioctyl), and Normax, a capsule combining danthron with docusate, work on the same principle. Agiolax combines granules of senna with a bulking agent.

It is hard to choose between so many excellent products. Many patients have their own favourite and their choice should be respected. Our preference is for bran because it is a natural food and Senokot or Dorbanex because they are the most economical.

Faecal smearing

A most distressing disorder of bowel control is faecal smearing. Faeces get everywhere, in the bed, in the clothing, in the patient's hair, under his nails, all over the lavatory. The patient is without insight and denies that all this is anything to do with him.

People who behave in this way have faecal retention, faecal incontinence and brain damage. Some are attempting in a confused way to relieve their own faecal retention manually. When the bowel is kept clear in a more acceptable manner, the problem ceases. Others appear not to recognise faeces as faeces. With them kindness is all important. Reproaches will not help. They, too, may need to have the bowel cleared. They may then require a regime of regular enemas or suppositories.

Toilet facilities

It is important for the older patient to preserve the habit of going to the lavatory. He is much more likely to remain continent if he has ready access to suitable toilet facilities. Old people need the lavatory more often than younger patients and they stay there longer.

In hospital one WC to every four patients and a commode to every bed should be the standard. The lavatories should not all be in one place. Some must be near the wards and bathrooms, others near the dayrooms including the physiotherapy, occupational therapy and dining areas. In a day hospital there should be a lavatory near the entrance. Lavatories must have level access. There should be no steps. The room must be warm, well lit and equipped with a call system. A wash basin must be near at hand, but not so placed as to make access difficult for wheelchair users. There is no reason why the lavatory should not be attractively decorated. In a well-designed building it should be possible for the patient to be within 10 m (33 ft) of a lavatory at all times.

The lavatory

Infirm old people need plenty of room in the lavatory. They are likely to be using a walking aid and perhaps a wheelchair. Some of them will be accompanied by a nurse. So at least one of the lavatories should be spacious, about 1.5 ×2 m (5 ×6.5 ft). In these larger rooms the WC should be placed off centre so that it can be approached from the side. Both right and left hand arrangements will be needed. There should be toilet paper on each side of the pan. The door must be wide enough to admit a wheelchair. If a patient falls it is easier to get to him if the door opens outwards, but this raises hazards for others who may be passing. Sliding doors or ones with double hinges may be a better solution, though unfamiliar at first to old people. Lavatory doors should be identifiable by a distinctive colour or an easily read sign. There must be a lock which can be opened from the outside in an emergency.

The WC should stand at least 30 cm (1 ft) from the back wall. Some patients, particularly double amputees, find it easier to sit astride the toilet facing the back wall. A high cistern gives more transfer space and a low one gives something to lean against.

A WC 45 mm (18 in) high suits most people. For those who need it, principally patients with stiff hips, the seat can be raised in a number of ways. The WC itself can be built up on a pedestal. A raised toilet seat, made of wood or plastic can be fitted or a frame holding a raised seat can stand over it (Fig. 55a). A raised seat generally makes the toilet unsuitable for a sanitary chair.

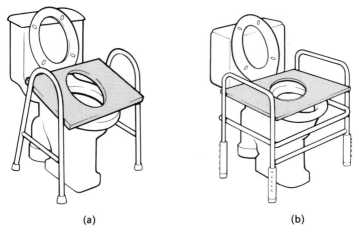

(a)   (b)

Fig. 55 (a) St. Helen's raised toilet frame with sloping seat is convenient for patients with stiff hips
    (b) Adjustable height toilet seat and frame

Handrails

Handrails are essential. A horizontal rail at a height of about 80 cm (32 in) from the door to the WC and continued alongside it is helpful. So is a vertical rail, wall mounted or fixed from floor to ceiling about 30 cm (12 in) in front of the WC (Fig. 56a). With off centre WCs these rails should be on one side only to facilitate transfer from the other side. An additional horizontal rail behind the lavatory may be helpful. Other lavatories can do with simpler arrangements. Wall-mounted sloping rails running upwards and away from the WC suit many people (Fig. 56b). Alternatively a toilet frame may be placed around the WC. This can be fixed to the floor or free standing. Some models incorporate a raised toilet seat and are of

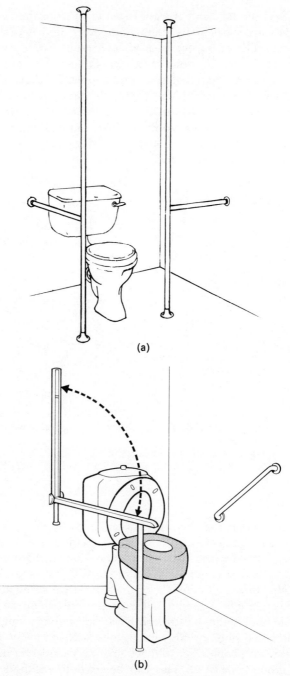

(a)

(b)

Fig. 56 a, b

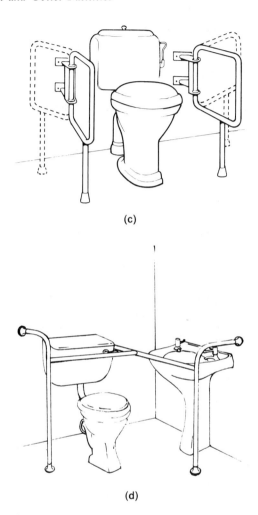

(c)

(d)

Fig. 56 Handrails
    (a) Vertical toilet rails
    (b) Sloping wall rail and Renray upward hingeing rail
    (c) Renray cloverleaf rails
    (d) DHSS recommended rails for lavatory and washbasin, ref. 33/68

adjustable height (Fig. 55b). There are situations in which it is convenient to have toilet rails which can be folded out of the way. The Renray Cloverleaf folds sideways against the wall but requires a lot of space on either side of the WC (Fig. 56c). Where space is restricted the Renray model, which hinges upwards against the back wall, though not very rigid, is a possible solution (Fig. 56b). In a large toilet for wheelchair users there is much to be said for the arrangement of rails recommended by the Government for the use of the disabled in public lavatories (Fig. 56d).

Mecanaids toilet aid

It is reassuring to a frail patient to have something to hold on to while sitting on the toilet. The Mecanaids toilet aid consists of two hinged arms which are fixed to the back of the lavatory and swing across the front of the user like the arms in a ski lift. They provide useful support for frail or unsteady patients (Fig. 57).

Sanitary chair

The patient who cannot walk to the lavatory can still get there in a sanitary chair. This is a toilet seat on wheels, by means of which the patient may move directly over the WC. The chair is very mobile and great care must be taken to prevent it moving at the wrong time. The sanitary chair affords the patient a measure of privacy which is very desirable. The nurse should not, however, use it merely to save time. If there is any possibility that the patient can walk to the lavatory he should do so.

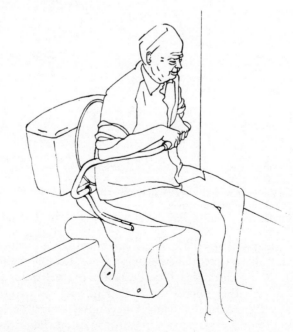

Fig. 57 Mecanaids toilet aid

Commodes

Commodes are made with various receptacles including a bedpan. Purpose made receptacles are more popular with patients because they are deeper. They are also easier to clean by hand. In hospital, however, where there is a bedpan washer the bedpan is more acceptable. A commode equipped with a detachable bedpan rack can be used as a sanitary chair if desired. If so it will have four wheels and these must be braked before it is left by a patient's bed.

Chemical closets

In hospital emptying a commode presents no problem. For an old person living alone and unable to get to the lavatory things are very different. In this situation a chemical closet, as used in caravans, is a useful solution. It may need emptying only once a week but when full it is very heavy. The chemicals may have a pervasive smell but the treated contents are not offensive and can be emptied down the lavatory. The Hassa commode is well designed and includes an adjustable height facility. It can also fold like a suitcase which makes it convenient for transportation.

Getting on and off the commode

At the stage when he needs a commode the patient is probably still in need of some help. The nurse should be familiar with the ways in which she can best assist him. One good method is to help the patient to his feet, remove his chair and replace it with the commode. Unless the patient can stand alone or with a walking aid this method needs two nurses. One supports him while the other moves the chair. Alternatively the commode can be placed alongside the patient's chair. This is suitable only if the patient can take a step or two and if both chair and commode stand against a wall so that they cannot slip.

It is often better, however, to place the commode at right angles to the chair. The patient is then helped to his feet and pivots round to the commode. This method gives the nurse more control. She can place her foot behind the chair leg and so prevent it from slipping as the patient gets up. In the same way she can steady the commode as he sits down. Whichever method is used the patient should be taught to feel for the arms of the chair or commode before sitting down. Once he is seated the commode can be moved to face the bedside. This reduces the danger of the patient falling forwards. He should be given privacy by the use of screens or curtains.

For further reading:

BROCKLEHURST, J. C. (Ed). 1985. *Textbook of Geriatric Medicine and Gerontology*, 3rd edition. Edinburgh: Churchill Livingstone.

For toilet equipment, hand rails, etc. *see* the catalogues of the Disabled Living Foundation and various manufacturers, especially Carters, Mecanaids and Renray Limited.

20
The Patient with Mental Impairment

One of the most characteristic features of a ward for elderly people is the large number of patients with mental as well as physical disturbance.

The mental disturbances of the elderly have been the subject of much research in recent years. It is known that 20 per cent of people over 80 living at home have some degree of mental impairment, about half of them to a severe degree. In an acute geriatric ward approximately one-third of the patients may be mentally impaired. In a long-stay ward the number will be much higher. Every nurse will become familiar with these problems and see them as a normal part of the older patient's care.

Organic and functional

Mental disturbances in old age are classified as organic or functional, though in practice both kinds of illness are often present in the same patient. Multiple pathology is as common in the mental sphere as it is in the physical.

Organic disorders are those caused by physical changes in the structure of the brain. Functional disorders are emotional and behavioural changes which may occur in patients whose brains are perfectly normal, though they also often accompany organic mental illness. Every individual is different and each patient's reaction to his illness, mental or physical, is coloured by his personality.

Brain failure

Organic mental illness is now often known as brain failure. This puts it on a par with other forms of organ failure, heart failure, respiratory failure or renal failure, ideas which nurses and doctors have been familiar with for generations. Brain failure may be acute or chronic. As in the case of an acute exacerbation of chronic bronchitis, acute on chronic brain failure is commonly seen in the older patient.

Acute brain failure

Acute brain failure may occur in those who are previously normal in mind, but it is commoner when the patient already has some mental impairment. Other predisposing factors include deafness, poor eyesight, Parkinson's disease and alcoholism. Acute brain failure may occur as a single incident, or as recurrent attacks of confusion and restlessness, often at night. Characteristically the situation fluctuates. Acute brain failure corresponds to the delirium which is seen in severe illness at any age. In the elderly it is more easily provoked.

Causes of acute brain failure

Psychological factors such as the effect of unfamiliar surroundings, frustration and depression, play some part in the development of acute brain failure, but physical factors are of greater importance.

An important cause is failure of the oxygen supply to the brain. This may result from heart failure, respiratory failure or anaemia. Acute infections are an important cause, especially pneumonia and urinary infections. Metabolic upsets, including dehydration, renal failure and diabetes (especially hypoglycaemia), may provoke acute brain failure. So may surgical operations, fractures and head injuries. Drugs are another important cause, especially sleeping tablets, the drugs used in Parkinsonism and antidepressants.

In some patients acute brain failure appears to be provoked by discomfort, particularly when the patient has an over full bowel or bladder. An examination of these organs is one of the first steps in the assessment of a patient who suddenly becomes confused.

A patient with acute brain failure is restless, anxious, and often noisy. At times he may seem quite lucid and at other times angry or frightened. He may fail to realise where he is, what time it is or who are the people around him. He may fail to recognise his friends and relations. He misinterprets what he sees and may resist the attentions of the nurse. He is often worse at night and is indeed living in a kind of nightmare. His speech may be rambling and incoherent. He is very likely to want to get out of bed.

Care of the patient with acute brain failure

The patient should, if possible, be nursed in a side ward as he is likely to disturb the rest of the ward. It is then possible to leave the light on, which he may find a comfort. The patient who becomes disturbed at night will cause the nurse much anxiety but as she gains experience she will acquire confidence which will reassure him. She should speak gently but firmly. She should explain repeatedly where he is, who she is and what is being done. If he tries to get out of bed she should not argue with him or restrain him with cot sides but should ensure that the bed is in a low position so that he may get out safely. It is best to help him into a chair or to take him to the lavatory. He can then be offered a cup of tea or even something stronger.

The patient is often seriously ill and the best way to control acute brain failure is to give the proper treatment for the disease which provoked it. It is also important to give sufficient fluid to prevent dehydration, not less than two litres a day. Some sedation is likely to be needed to prevent the restless patient from exhausting himself, the other patients in the ward, or those who are caring for him at home.

Outcome of acute brain failure

Some patients with acute brain failure recover their mental equilibrium within a day or two or even a few hours. Others, especially those with severe physical illness, may die. Others again, may pass into a state of permanent dementia. Any pre-existing mental impairment is likely to be made worse.

Chronic brain failure (dementia)

Chronic brain failure or dementia is characterised by permanent mental impairment. This may be of mild, moderate or severe degree. It is always due to damage to the structure of the brain.

Causes of chronic brain failure

Much the commonest cause of chronic brain failure after the age of 75 is loss of brain cells. This is currently known as Senile Dementia Alzheimer Type (SDAT). The changes are similar to those described in Alzheimer's disease, a form of dementia occurring in younger patients.

In a few patients, often those with previous hypertension, dementia occurs as a result of repeated small strokes with cumulative damage to the brain. This is known as multi-infarct dementia.

Dementia may also be a feature of patients with cerebral tumour, normal pressure hydrocephalus, alcoholism and Parkinson's disease.

Senile dementia Alzheimer type (SDAT)

In a patient with SDAT the onset of brain failure is gradual. The old person may relinquish his former interest in life, give up his hobbies and lose his initiative, but the outstanding feature is his failure of memory. He forgets first what has happened recently. His memory for distant events lasts longer and he may appear to live in the past. He may be able to preserve a social facade, concealing the gaps in his memory by fabrication, a process known as confabulation. Forgetfulness may proceed to the point where the patient fails to recognise people he knows well. He may mistake his daughter or even the nurse for his mother. At some point in this process he may become depressed.

The progressive failure of memory renders the old person incompetent. A woman leaves the kettle on until it boils dry or forgets to light the gas. She forgets to shop, to clean, even to change her clothes. Her home and her person become increasingly dirty. A man forgets to shave, to fasten his fly buttons and does not notice when he has spilled food on his clothing. Forgetfulness also leads to deterioration in toilet habits. The old person may forget to go to the lavatory and become incontinent. A man may pass water against a wall or into a waste paper basket, mistaking these for the lavatory. After an accident with the bowels an old lady may conceal her faeces in a drawer. In those who become faecally impacted faecal smearing may occur.

Disorientation in space

A further consequence of forgetfulness is disorientation in space. The patient may wander away from home and be unable to find the way back or to tell anyone his address. He may forget the way about his house. He loses his belongings and then may accuse others of stealing them.

Disorientation in time

He may also become disorientated in time. He forgets when to go to bed and when to get up. The rhythm of his sleep is disturbed and he may upset the household by wandering about at night. Such nocturnal restlessness is often the prelude to an acute incident of confusion, requiring hospital treatment.

Judgement

Failure of memory also impairs the old person's judgement. He becomes irresponsible, making unnecessary purchases, giving money away on impulse or failing to pay his bills.

Personality

In addition an old person may deteriorate in his personality and become more self-centred. He may lose his powers of self-criticism and self-control, his awareness of the needs of others. He may become irritable, awkward or even aggressive making life intolerable for those he lives with. Yet he is without insight into the problems he is creating and blames others for every difficulty which may provoke a crisis with his family or neighbours. This is not bound to happen, however, and some people remain pleasantly confused. Much depends on their previous personality and emotional stability.

Physical change

Physically the patient may become weaker. He may develop a shuffling gait and falls are common. Such patients can usually be managed in a general hospital.

Wandering

The greatest problems arise when mental deterioration outruns the physical. The robust old person with a tendency to wander is most difficult to handle. He may need care in a specialist residential home or psychiatric hospital.

Course of SDAT

The patient with SDAT is likely to become gradually worse but the pace of his decline is variable. In some people the illness never amounts to much more than chronic absentmindedness, and the rest of the patient's personality is well preserved. In others the decline is rapid, especially when the old person is isolated from social contact by failure of sight and hearing, bereavement, rejection or physical handicap. A patient who begins to dement in his 60s or early 70s often becomes more severely disabled than one whose brain begins to fail after the age of 75.

The patient often comes to hospital because of an acute confusional episode, a fall, an intercurrent infection or a social crisis provoked by illness in his principal supporter. About half of those admitted to hospital die within three months.

Multi-infarct dementia (vascular brain failure)

Multi-infarct dementia or vascular brain failure results from impairment of the blood supply to the brain. In other words it is mental impairment resulting from little strokes. It is thus frequently associated with other manifestations of stroke illness, such as hemiplegia, disturbances of speech and vision and pseudo-bulbar palsy. Many of the patients suffer from hypertension. The age of onset is commonly a few years earlier than in SDAT. There are, however, many mixed cases where the features of SDAT and multi-infarct dementia are combined.

Clinical features of multi-infarct dementia. Multi-infarct dementia is likely to begin with a minor stroke from which the patient fails to make a complete recovery. Because the brain damage is patchy the patient's judgement and basic personality may be fairly well preserved. He may, for the same reason, retain rather more insight than is common in primary brain failure. He is, therefore, more likely to become depressed when he realises what is happening to him. In the later stages of multi-infarct dementia many patients become cheerful, noisy, aggressive, incontinent or withdrawn. Because of their associated physical infirmity most of these patients are cared for in general hospital or nursing homes.

Course of multi-infarct dementia. In contrast to the steady decline of many patients with SDAT, the downhill course of the patient with multi-infarct dementia is marked by a series of incidents. Each one represents a further small cerebral infarct or little stroke and is followed by partial recovery. This is often enough to enable a patient recently admitted to hospital to be discharged again, but he never quite regains his former level. Sometimes the course of the illness is punctuated by epileptic fits or by episodes of acute or chronic brain failure.

Treatment of the dementing patient

There are no drugs which have a direct effect on the dementing process and the fewer drugs old people take the better, especially when their memory is unreliable. If the patient is restless, however, a tranquilliser, perhaps haloperidol, may help. If he is depressed an antidepressant is given, preferably at night. Many drugs are promoted in an effort to improve the function of the failing brain, for example isoxsuprine (Duvadilan), cyclandelate (Cyclospasmol), naftidrofuryl (Praxilene) and co-dergocrine mesylate (Hydergine). All these drugs may lead to minor improvements but none alters the clinical picture decisively.

If night sedation is needed chlormethiazole (Heminevrin) and chloral (Noctec) or its derivatives are the safest hypnotics. Many of the benzodiazepines, for example the short-acting temazepam (Euhypnos, Normison) or lormetazepam (Noctamid) are preferred to the longer-acting drugs like nitrazepam (Mogadon) because of the absence of hangover effects in the morning.

Management and nursing care

Drugs are of limited value to the patient with brain failure. Success lies rather in good management. If possible the old person should remain in his own home with the support of his family, his general practitioner and the domiciliary services. The burden of anxiety and sheer hard work on his carers is often very great. The situation may be eased by regular day care and periodic respite admissions to hospital or a residential home. Community psychiatric nurses (CPN) have a special responsibility to keep in touch with families and offer support to carers when necessary. In this way the patient's quality of life is enhanced and his carers are helped before they reach breaking point. Such timely assistance is the best way of preventing neglect or abuse of the elderly patient. Even though the patient's disease has no cure, the emotional and social problems can be made more bearable.

In hospital

In hospital the aim is to introduce the patient to an environment where he can feel at home and establish easy relationships with the staff. They must be able to accept the patient for what he is without becoming irritated or trying to change his ways. His individuality must be respected and he must feel that he has a say in what is happening to him. If a patient is hostile the nurse should ask herself whether she did anything to provoke him. Did she perhaps fail to give him sufficient explanation? The patient who is most difficult is often the one who is in greatest need of reassurance. Mentally impaired old people remain sensitive to the emotional atmosphere and will respond only to a person who approaches them with tact and kindness.

Reality orientation (RO)

It is important for the staff to keep the patient in touch with reality and to build up his sense of identity. This is the basis of the technique of reality orientation (RO). The patient should be addressed by name, his first name or surname as he prefers. This is easier if he wears a name badge like the staff. He should have his name on his locker and he should have some of his belongings with him. His bed should be readily identifiable. Clocks and calendars should be in evidence to help his sense of orientation in time.

Communication

Every opportunity should be taken by the staff to sit down with the patient and converse, both being at the same level so that eye contact can be maintained. Touch helps express friendliness and concern, as well as engaging the patient's attention. The nurse should therefore be ready to hold the patient's hand.

Communication is made easier if the patient's spectacles are clean so that he can see who he is talking to, his hearing aid is working and his dentures in place.

All this helps to build up the patient's sense of his identity and worth. Choice, too, is important. The patient should have an opportunity to decide what he will wear. His food preferences should be consulted. If he never eats fish or has special religious or cultural dietary requirements, that fact should be remembered. Food can be offered with a question, 'Would you like some of these carrots?' Food should be taken at a table so that the patient is aware of his companions and only one course should be offered at a time.

Ward routine

Mentally impaired old people lose their initiative and they cannot remember what to do next. Habit is the best prop and, if they are in hospital, ward routines assume an important place in their life. The regular events of the day, getting up, washing, dressing, going to toilet, meals and occupational therapy form an ordered framework to the patient's life. They give him a sense of security. Conversely a change in routine or of environment can upset him completely. It is important to allow the patient plenty of time. In a busy ward this is easier said than done, but old people cannot be hurried. If pressed too hard they may exhibit a catastrophic reaction, becoming muddled, irritable, incontinent and refusing to try further.

The patient may need help in the activities of living and it is important to maintain his dignity. He needs privacy for dressing and toilet. However, single rooms, even if available, are seldom desirable for the patient with severe brain failure. He is more likely to find security in company.

Restlessness

Some patients with mental impairment are prepared to lie in bed or sit in a chair all day in a state of apathy and inactivity. This is especially likely if they are on large doses of hypnotics or tranquillisers. Such patients will sleep better at night and require fewer drugs if they can be kept active during the day.

Other patients, however, may exhibit restlessness and indulge in purposeless over-activity. In some cases this may take the form of wandering. If a patient is wandering the nurse should avoid a confrontation. She should try to divert his attention rather than restrain him. 'Are you looking for the lavatory?' or 'Will you come and help me lay the table?' are better than 'Why don't you sit down?'

Patients who are inclined to wander should not be locked in. They seldom make determined efforts to pass through a door which does not open easily. An additional handle high up on the door above eye level will restrain them. In another form of over-activity the patient, usually a woman, may turn out her locker, luggage or handbag with repeated packing and unpacking. She is probably hunting for something but cannot remember what. She may not recognise her own property and this may lead to difficulty with other patients. Once again distraction and alternative occupation is the answer.

Restless patients should never be restrained in a geriatric chair with a tray across the front. This will only increase their frustration and distress.

Activities

In hospital the occupational therapist uses many different techniques which the nurse and other carers can practise also. Art work, especially collage, and other crafts give a sense of achievement. The things that the patients have made should be displayed in the ward. Some very confused old people will make articles of surprisingly high quality if they are given the right opportunity. Because of their lack of initiative, however, they should work under close supervision and they need help quickly when they get into difficulties.

Domestic activities, including preparation of food, table laying and the washing and drying of dishes, all recall to women skills which once gave status and satisfaction. They provoke interest and discussion in a group and make the individual feel more at home. Games like dominoes, bingo and quizzes produce great enthusiasm but not all patients like them. Those who wish to opt out should be allowed to do so. Music is popular, particularly hymns and old time songs. Some confused patients can enjoy playing in a percussion band. Patients vary greatly in their response to radio and television. Some enjoy them greatly, others are irritated, bored or bewildered. It is better to use broadcasting for a purpose than as a background noise.

Pictures may give great satisfaction. They stimulate reminiscence. Some old people can be happy for hours, day after day, sorting through picture postcards and family photographs. The outside world remains of interest, and outings are always popular, not only for the event itself but also because of the discussion and conversation it provokes. Even when they cannot get out, patients enjoy watching the passing scene from the window and discussing what they see.

A ward for mentally disturbed old people should have a regular programme of activities. This should be displayed on the wall for all to see (see p. 81).

Occupational therapy

The nurse and the occupational therapist have much to learn from each other. Between them they can work wonders by recreating in the old person a sense of his dignity as a human being.

Problems such as wandering are best managed by getting the patient to do something more constructive. This is why occupational therapy is so important. It is not enough to keep old people warm, clean and fed. They should lead creative lives as far as their failing powers permit. The occupational therapist not only provides interesting things for the patient to do, but she draws them together in a group so that they take more notice of each other. Such a group acquires a kind of collective emotion and if the atmosphere has been a happy one the patient will be more content and the nurses' work more enjoyable.

For further reading:

HOLDEN, U. & WOODS, R. 1982. *Reality Orientation*. Edinburgh: Churchill Livingstone.

LAY, C. & WOODS, R. 1984. *Caring for the Person with Dementia*. Alzheimer's Disease Society.

LEVY, R. & POST, F. 1982. *Psychiatry of Late Life*. Oxford: Blackwell.

NORMAN, A. 1982. *Mental Illness in Old Age*. Centre for Policy on Ageing.

21

The Patient with Emotional Disturbance

Dementia is an organic disorder caused by changes in the structure of the brain. Equally common in the older patient are emotional disturbances which do not result from structural changes in the brain. These are known as functional disorders.

Functional and organic disturbances are contrasted for the purposes of teaching, but it is important to understand that they often occur together in the same patient at the same time. The principal functional disorder of late life is depressive illness.

Depressive illness

Depressive illness affects at least 5 out of every 100 persons living in the community. It is as common as brain failure in extreme old age and is the principal mental illness of those between 60 and 75. Depressive illness is the source of much misery and may lead to suicide. The symptoms differ only in intensity and duration from the unhappiness which everyone experiences in misfortune or grief. For this reason depressive illness may be overlooked in the older patient, exposed as he is to physical illness, bereavement, loneliness, poverty and the sense that he is a burden to others.

Loss, it has been said, is the principal theme of depression in old age. Problems are likely to be multiple and the older and less adaptable the patient the more likely he is to have to face new losses. Depressive illness seems to occur in those who are predisposed to it by heredity and by their approach to life. Some take the trials of old age in their stride but others are unable to do so.

Cause of depressive illness. As with most mental illness, depression has no single cause. It probably results from an interaction between the events of the patient's life, his physical health, and his inherited constitution. In more than half the patients who suffer from depression in old age there is serious concomitant physical illness. In a few cases drugs contribute also. Reserpine and methyldopa, used for the treatment of hypertension, and phenobarbitone used for the treatment of epilepsy, are well known examples.

Reactive depression

When a patient's depression seems to be largely determined by unhappy experiences like bereavement, loneliness or physical illness it is spoken of as reactive or situational depression. In people of neurotic temperament the term neurotic depression is also used. In geriatric wards this type of depression is a common response to the many severe and disabling illnesses which affect the older patient. It is especially likely to occur in people with malignant disease, heart failure or stroke. It is probably a normal phase in the process of dying. Depression may co-exist with other forms of mental illness, particularly the early stages of brain failure when the patient still retains insight and is aware of his diminishing powers.

Patients with reactive depression may have difficulty in getting to sleep. Their mood is often worse in the evening, but it may lift relatively easily. The patient does not usually lose weight.

Endogenous depression

Where external circumstances play little part and a change in the patient's emotions has no obvious cause, the illness is often described as endogenous or psychotic depression. In such cases heredity plays an important role. There is often a history of depressive illness or mania in earlier life. There may be a family history of depression also.

Endogenous depression is characterised by early morning waking. The patient wakes in the small hours and may fail to go to sleep again. In the morning he feels at his worst but his mood may lighten a little in the evening. He may lose appetite and weight.

The Spectrum of Depressive Illness

Endogenous and reactive depression are not hard and fast alternatives. Rather they should be thought of as opposite ends of a spectrum. There will be some features which are reactive and some which are endogenous, but the proportion will vary in each individual.

Clinical features of the depressed patient

A depressive illness has a fairly clear beginning. The patient or his relatives can usually remember when he ceased to be himself. His change of mood may range from mild loss of interest in life to total despair with tearfulness and thoughts of suicide. The patient's mood often varies with the time of day. Quite often sadness is not obvious but the patient is anxious, worried or irritable. Occasionally he may conceal his real feelings behind a mask of assumed cheerfulness. The patient may be troubled by a sense of inadequacy or guilt. He tends to withdraw from social contacts which he formerly enjoyed. He may become deluded and believe that he has committed an unforgivable crime or sin. Such feelings increase the risk of suicide.

The patient with endogenous depression may exhibit retardation with slowness of thought and movement. He is unable to make decisions, and tasks which he once took in his stride become too much for him. More often though his misery is accompanied by agitation and restlessness.

Physical symptoms

A depressed patient may suffer with morbid concern about his body. His symptoms may mimic almost any physical disease. Loss of energy, constipation, a sense of pressure in the head, difficulty in swallowing, breathlessness or bizarre pains may be the principal manifestations of his illness. He may lose his appetite and have a disturbed sense of taste. He may take refuge in alcohol, drugs or compulsive eating. His sleep pattern is commonly disturbed.

A patient with physical illness may fail to respond to medical treatment and rehabilitation. A person who has a stroke, or heart attack or who suffers from Parkinson's disease, may not make the progress expected, and often depressive illness will prove to be the reason.

Depressed or demented?

A depressed patient may have periods of confusion and appear to be demented. He may feel so hopeless that he becomes forgetful and unable to concentrate. He will then get a low score on mental testing. If such a patient is recognised and given treatment for depressive illness his apparent brain failure will disappear like magic.

Treatment of the depressed patient

The patient who is severely depressed is usually treated in a mental hospital but such patients represent only the tip of the iceberg. For every depressed patient admitted to a mental hospital there are fifteen who never see a psychiatrist but are treated by their general practitioner, geriatrician, or other doctors. Perhaps ten times as many never consult a doctor at all. In old age a great deal of depression results from physical illness. In addition to the treatment for his physical disabilities the patient needs to feel that somebody understands him as a person and can sympathise with his sense of hopelessness and worry. He must never be told to snap out of it or to pull himself together. Such advice only makes him worse.

Depressed patients are isolated by their misery and need to be drawn back into the community. If they are inpatients, life on the ward can help them. If they are outpatients, the day hospital aims to achieve the same effect. A kind and welcoming staff offering treatment and recreation in a friendly atmosphere can do much to lift the spirits of the depressed old person.

Personal problems also contribute to depressive illness. The struggle to survive in an uncaring world may have proved too much. Bereavement or unhappy relationships may also have played a part. In all this, the social worker is the expert. She will help the patient to come to terms with his problems and may be able to suggest practical help. Many patients can be assisted by these measures but some also need drugs.

Drug treatment

Drugs available for the treatment of depression in the older patient fall into two major groups, the antidepressants and lithium. There is a third group, the monoamine-oxidase inhibitors (MAOI), but these have serious side effects and the patient must observe various dietary restrictions. For these reasons they are seldom prescribed for the older patient.

Tricyclic and related antidepressants. The antidepressant drugs include imipramine (Tofranil) and amitriptyline (Tryptizol). All antidepressants have some sedative action. This is stronger in amitriptyline which is normally given to the patient with anxiety and agitation. Imipramine is a weaker sedative and is preferred for the patient who is retarded. Because of the sedative action antidepressant drugs are usually given at night in place of sleeping tablets.

The most serious side effect of antidepressants is postural hypotension which causes dizziness, faints and falls. These drugs may also cause confusion, particularly in patients who already have a mild degree of brain failure. The other side effects resemble those of atropine. They include a dry mouth, constipation, difficulty in visual accommodation, retention of urine and tremor. Antidepressants may have to be avoided in patients with glaucoma or prostatic disease because they make these troubles worse. But in spite of the side effects the tricyclic drugs and those related to them are extremely useful and provide the mainstay of treatment for depressive illness.

Every year sees new antidepressants brought on to the market. None is more effective than the original drugs imipramine and amitriptyline. The new drugs are inevitably much more expensive but they are less likely to cause side effects.

Depressed patients often show response to treatment within a week but it is necessary to persevere for a month before deciding that a drug does not work. If one does not work it is always worth trying another. One patient in five will fail to respond to antidepressant drugs. Once treatment is established it is normally continued for six months or longer if there is a tendency to relapse.

Lithium. Lithium carbonate (Camcolit) or the sustained release preparation Priadel, was originally used for the treatment of mania. Later it was found to help people with depression especially those prone to recurrent attacks. The dose must be carefully monitored to keep the level in the blood between 0.5 and 1.5 mmol/l. Overdosage causes tremor, confusion, vomiting and diarrhoea. The necessity for frequent blood tests restricts its usefulness.

Other drugs. Depressed patients whose agitation is not controlled by antidepressant medication may also need an additional tranquilliser. If they need a sleeping drug, and they often do, it should be one with which suicide is impossible. The benzodiazepines are suitable. Barbiturates should be avoided at all costs.

Course of depressive illness

Many patients with reactive depression associated with physical illness recover quickly. As their health improves they discover that there is still something to live for, especially if their social circumstances can be made easier at the same time.

But the severely depressed patient whose illness has a large endogenous component does not do so well. Only one in three recover completely. In over half the illness is likely to run a relapsing course. In the remainder there may be no response to treatment.

Neurosis

Old age with its many stresses and trials is the ultimate test of personality. Some people, perhaps predisposed by heredity, develop neuroses with symptoms of morbid anxiety. Anxiety in a situation of acute stress like an examination is normal, but prolonged and inappropriate anxiety, out of all proportion to the cause, is pathological and is called an anxiety state. Some 10 per cent of old people suffer in this way. About half develop their symptoms in old age. The others bring their neuroses with them from earlier life. Women are more often affected than men. The borderline between an anxiety state and a depression is tenuous since prolonged anxiety can itself be a cause of neurotic depression and there is a good deal of overlap.

Some neurotic patients complain of anxiety, worry or nerves but most express their fears in a host of physical symptoms. The patient may complain of chest pain, palpitations, faintness or breathlessness giving rise to fears of heart disease. Dysphagia, abdominal pain and bowel disturbance may suggest the possibility of cancer. Headaches and dizziness raise fears of a cerebral tumour. Forgetfulness, failure of concentration and irritability make the patient wonder if he is going mad. Muscular tension anywhere in the body may provoke obscure pains which demand investigation. With or without these symptoms the patient may be chronically tired. He may have difficulty getting to sleep and wake exhausted in the mornings. He may lose appetite and weight. The patient who constantly expresses his emotional conflicts and his dissatisfaction with life in these ways may become preoccupied with his health to the exclusion of all other interests. He is then known as a hypochondriac.

With physical disease of all kinds commoner in old age than at any other time of life, there is a great deal of interaction between the patient's physical and mental state. A factor which lowers his resistance to neurosis and makes his anxiety symptoms worse may indeed be a new physical illness. When an old person develops anxiety symptoms for the first time in late life or a chronic anxiety state becomes worse the doctor will look very carefully for a new physical reason.

Treatment of the neurotic patient

Neurosis itself is seldom a reason for admission to the hospital, though the nurse will meet plenty of patients with physical disease who also have neurotic personalities. Anxiety can often be relieved if it is freely expressed. A careful history and physical examination by the doctor followed by explanation and reassurance is itself therapeutic. The social worker with her insight into human relationships can help the patient come to terms with his problems and interpret them to other members of the team. The nurses and therapist can offer support by listening with understanding to what the patient has to say and by encouraging him to participate in the life of the ward. Group activity draws the patient out of himself and thus helps him to see his own troubles in perspective.

Drug treatment relies principally on tranquillisers. Diazepam (Valium) is one of the best. Oxazepam (Serenid D) and chlordiazepoxide (Librium) are also widely prescribed. Tranquillisers alleviate the patient's anxieties but are much more effective when accompanied by explanation, reassurance and a genuine interest in his problems. Patients who are depressed as well as anxious will need one of the antidepressants described above.

Paranoid illness

Some old people are unreasonably suspicious and suffer from a sense of persecution. These are the central features of paranoid illness. A paranoid patient may be deluded, believing what is not true, or hallucinated, hearing or seeing things that are not there. He is often hostile to those around him. He may accuse them of trying to harm him, perhaps by poisoning his food or stealing his possessions. Paranoid symptoms do not necessarily indicate a specific illness. They may occur in all forms of mental disturbance, including acute confusion, dementia and depression. An old person isolated by deafness or physical handicap is particularly likely to be affected.

One small group of patients with persecutory symptoms stand out from the rest. They suffer from late paraphrenia, the schizophrenia of old age. The patient with late paraphrenia is usually a woman living alone. Earlier in life she may have been eccentric, arrogant or suspicious. She may believe that her neighbours have sexual designs on her, are spying on her or directing harmful rays against her. Yet in spite of this her personality remains intact. She does not become disorientated or lose touch with her surroundings. She may be able to discuss topics other than her delusions quite sensibly. She is likely to be in fair physical health and may survive for many years.

Treatment of paranoid patients

Paranoid patients require prolonged treatment. Phenothiazines help them most. Trifluoperazine (Stelazine) and thioridazine (Melleril) are the best. For those who will not take tablets or medicines the long-acting fluphenazine (Moditen) can be used. Most patients do well, provided an adequate dose is maintained permanently. This inevitably risks side effects, particularly Parkinsonism, and drugs may have to be given to control this. If the patient has someone to care for him he may live at home for a long time. If isolated he may need residential care. In a crisis he may have to come to hospital.

These patients, with their suspicious natures and delusions of persecution, are particularly difficult for the nurse to handle. They are likely to provoke in her, as in the rest of society, feelings of hostility and rejection which can only make matters worse. Their delusions must be accepted with sympathy and without criticism. The skilled nurse, because of her own inner certainty and training may be able to make such patients feel secure. If so their hostility will diminish and they will become happier and easier to manage.

Personality disorder

Every individual is different and each patient's reaction to his illness is coloured by his personality. Old age removes the mask of inhibition by which people make themselves acceptable to others, but at the same time it makes them more dependent. If a person has never got on well with others, problems are more likely when he is old and in need of care.

There are some people, probably about 3 per cent of the elderly, whose difficulties in human relationships justify a diagnosis of personality disorder. They are life's misfits. Warped, cantankerous, belligerent, they have a talent for antagonising those who might otherwise help them. Such people may, of course, become physically ill, demented or depressed but nothing will alter their personality. They remain the people they always were. Their personality defects are not a mental illness and they may be people of high intelligence. Sometimes they have a record of conflict with the law, but in old age shoplifting and rather pathetic sexual offences are likely to be their only misdemeanours. Others are eccentric, inadequate or alcoholic, drifting down the social scale to end in isolation and squalor. They may be understandably rejected by their relatives. Intelligent eccentrics who live in squalor are said to exhibit Diogenes syndrome. The name comes from an ancient Greek philosopher who made a virtue of living in discomfort.

Such people are unlikely to be on good terms with their general practitioner and may have been struck off his list. When they are ill they may find their way to hospital via the casualty department. Once in they may be demanding towards the staff. Since personality disorder is part of a person's character and not a disease it is unrealistic to look for a cure, and drugs are needed only for associated illness. As with those who are demented the aim must be to accept the patient for what he is. At the same time it may have to be made clear that other people also have their rights.

Patients are not admitted to hospital primarily because of a personality disorder. Admission is required only if they need care and treatment for some physical disease. They may have no proper home and their resettlement demands all the skill of the social worker. A few will need continuing care in hospital. They do not always create the problems that might be expected if the atmosphere of the ward is friendly and relaxed. If they do not fit into one ward they can be tried in another but too many moves may increase the patient's feelings of insecurity and rejection.

For further reading:

PITT, B. M. N. 1982. *Psychogeriatrics*. Edinburgh: Churchill Livingstone.
STANWAY, A. 1982. *Overcoming Depression*. Feltham: Hamlyn.

22
The Patient with Impaired Sight and Hearing

One old person in four has some visual impairment and two-thirds of those registered blind are over 65. However, of these only one in twenty is totally blind, unable to tell light from dark. For every two persons registered blind there is another registered as partially sighted, unable to read ordinary print with glasses.

Old people and those who care for them have been too ready in the past to accept failing eyesight as an inevitable consequence of ageing. In practice a substantial number can be helped to see better. Some old people fear that using their eyes will make their eyesight worse and avoid reading and watching TV in order to rest the eyes. This is a fallacy. The eyes cannot be damaged in this way.

Environment

To see well is an important way of keeping in touch with the world and the environment of the ward should promote this. Good lighting is vital. Old people have smaller pupils than young people and need more light. Bedside as well as ceiling lights are necessary. Every ward should have a large clock in a prominent position and a wall calendar of the day at a time variety. Large print books should be available from the hospital library. There are draughts, dominoes and playing cards for the visually handicapped and the ward or occupational therapy department should have a supply. The ward should also have a few magnifying glasses, the sort held in the hand and the strip type which covers the line of print. A tape recorder will enable the patient to receive talking letters. These can be a great joy especially when the sender is in another part of the world and unable to visit.

Presbyopia

Many people have refractive errors and need glasses all their lives. But the commonest visual disturbance in old age is presbyopia, a failure of the eye to accommodate for close work. It is caused by hardening of the lens and begins in most people about the age of fifty. It can be corrected by reading glasses. It is important to ensure that the patient has his glasses with him in hospital and that they are clean and in good repair. Glasses should be reviewed every few years. They should be marked with the owner's name, on the frame and in the case. The identure kit can be used for this purpose as well as for marking dentures (see p. 173).

Gradual loss of vision

The eye is part of the body and, if it fails in old age, it fails from medical causes, in the same way as other functions of the body fail. Failure is always due to a medical cause, never to over-use, over-strain or wrong glasses. Several diseases interfere with vision and may eventually cause blindness.

Cataract

A cataract is due to an opacity in the lens of the eye. A person with cataract sees the world like a car driver looking through a dirty windscreen (Fig. 58b). However, cataracts can be removed and are usually now replaced by an artificial lens which gives excellent results, providing the retina at the back of the eye is healthy. But the nurse will meet a diminishing number of people operated on before lens implants became general. Such people were supplied with pebble lenses which restricted and distorted their field of vision. With such lenses everything is magnified and straight lines appear curved. An alternative to pebble lenses is contact lenses, but few old people can manage these successfully.

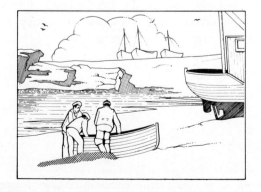

Fig. 58 a

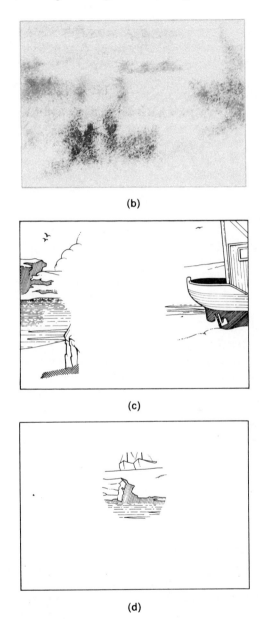

Fig. 58 (a) Normal vision

(b) 'Frosted glass' vision. The world as it appears to a patient with cataract

(c) Loss of central vision. The world as it appears to a patient with macular degeneration.

(d) Loss of peripheral vision. The world as it appears to a patient with glaucoma.

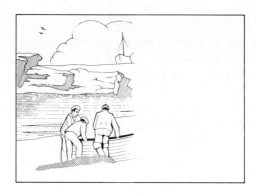

Fig. 58 (e) Loss of lateral vision. The world as it appears to a patient with hemianopia
A patient may suffer from more than one of these conditions at the same time.

Macular degeneration

Macular degeneration is the commonest cause of blindness in late life. It may occur by itself or be associated with cataract or other diseases of the eye. The cause is unknown, but in its early stages new blood vessels grow between the choroid and the retina, producing minute retinal detachments. Until recently there was no treatment for this, but now the advance of the disease can be halted by destroying the new blood vessels with a laser. Senile macular degeneration causes a serious loss of central vision but the patient can always see something out of the corner of his eye and can be reassured that he will not be plunged into total darkness (Fig. 58c).

Glaucoma

Glaucoma is characterised by increase of pressure within the eye and damage to the optic nerve. It may be quite painless. Unlike patients with macular degeneration those with glaucoma lose their peripheral field of vision. They may retain central vision for a long time, but to be able to see only straight ahead is a great disability (Fig. 58d). Some patients require surgical treatment. Others are kept going by eye drops such as pilocarpine and physostigmine which constrict the pupil and improve the flow of fluid within the eye. If the patient was using eye drops before he came to hospital, it is important that he should continue to do so in the ward.

Diabetes

Diabetes is also an important cause of visual loss in the elderly. It affects the lens and is one of the causes of cataract. It also involves the retina. Damage done by diabetes cannot be restored and there is doubt whether even strict management of the disease can prevent eye damage. But diabetic retinopathy, like macular degeneration, is associated with new blood vessel formation and can be treated by a laser.

Drug effects

Many drugs taken by the elderly may affect eyesight and a few can cause blindness. All drugs with an atropine-like action, for example antidepressants, tranquillisers and anti-Parkinsonian drugs, may cause blurring of vision and aggravate glaucoma. Steroids may predispose to cataract. Chloroquine used for the treatment of rheumatoid arthritis and ethambutol used for the treatment of tuberculosis may damage the retina.

Sudden loss of vision

To go blind gradually is bad enough but sudden loss of eyesight is catastrophic. The causes all relate to the blood supply of the eye. Thrombosis may occur in the central vein of the retina or in the central retinal artery. Cranial arteritis may also cause blindness. A partial visual loss, hemianopia, is a fairly common complication of a stroke. The patient loses one-half of his visual field and cannot see to one side. There is often a hemiplegia on the same side (Fig. 58e).

Recognition of blindness

Many old people who come to hospital for another reason have never been officially recognised as blind. It is not always apparent how little they can see and the nurse's observations may be of great value. A person does not have to be totally blind to qualify for the blind register, which carries considerable benefits, both financial and social. The patient, to qualify, must be 'blind within the meaning of the Act'. This implies a reduction of visual acuity or a restriction of visual field severe enough to prevent him from carrying out work for which eyesight is essential. The financial advantages of blind registration include increased income tax allowances, a reduced TV licence and free postage on items for the blind. Services for the blind include visiting, clubs, talking books, and the opportunity to learn

Braille or Moon. All this sustains the blind person's morale and helps him to face his handicap. The Royal National Institute for the Blind is a source of much helpful information as is the BBC's regular radio programme, 'In Touch'.

The person blinded in early life

The patient who has been blind for many years is usually well adjusted to his handicap. He has developed his memory and his other senses to make up for his lost eyesight. He has learned to find his way around, to identify objects by touch, to note carefully where he has put down his possessions so that he can find them again, to walk without groping, to read Braille or Moon. He has good contact with other people and his morale should not be in danger. If, however, he becomes deaf or infirm his handicaps are disproportionately increased and rehabilitation is harder.

The patient blinded in old age

The patient who has lost his eyesight in old age is in a much more difficult position. If he has gone blind suddenly he has suffered a shattering blow which may make him helpless, deeply depressed and possibly confused. If blindness comes on gradually he may find that his hearing, touch, balance and powers of learning are not sharp enough to compensate for his handicap. Such patients are naturally apprehensive and lack confidence. They run great risks of falling and this hinders their rehabilitation. Mercifully very few old people live in a world of total darkness. The majority who are blind within the meaning of the Act can see well enough to get about the house. Because they know their surroundingss so well they are much more confident there and if possible they should not be brought to hospital at all. Even in hospital, however, they are not bound to relapse into total dependency and the nurse must give them every encouragement to help themselves.

A blind person who is also mentally impaired often calls out for reassurance, as a baby cries to be picked up. His demands are distressing to other patients and to the staff. The best solution is to find someone, a relative, friend or volunteer, to sit with him.

Approaching the blind

The nurse, and anyone else who approaches a blind person, should introduce herself whenever she goes to him, so that he learns to recognise her voice. She should speak to him and touch him gently. She should never do anything for him without prior explanation. She should do all she can to help him adapt to his surroundings by teaching him the layout of the ward. She should be specially sensitive to his risk of tripping over an unfamiliar object. She should help him to arrange his possessions in identifiable places and can assist his dressing by putting out his clothes in the same order each day. When giving him food she should say what it is. Food may have to be cut up, but it need not be mixed up in a mush. The patient may have his own preference for a knife and fork or spoon and he should be allowed to choose. A plate bunker (see p. 134) is often of assistance. If the sight of one eye is better than the other, the nurse should see that the patient's locker and belongings are on the side with the better vision.

Helping the blind person to walk

Many blind people need guidance to walk and the staff must be prepared to escort them about the ward. When she does this the nurse should learn to offer her arm to the patient so that he takes her arm and not vice versa. In this way the patient will walk automatically a little behind her. This will give him confidence and some sense of direction and a feeling that things are not entirely outside his control. If a nurse takes his arm, she tends to propel him in front of her, which is bad for his self-confidence as he has no sense of where he is going. When approaching a chair, a blind person, like a sighted one, should reach for the arms with both hands and should feel the seat of the chair against the back of his legs before he sits down. A blind person will almost certainly need a walking stick and if unsteady may be better with a walking aid.

Outdoors a white stick warns other road users of the vulnerability of the person with a visual handicap. Anyone who guides such a person out of doors should approach steps and curves at right angles and not obliquely and should be prepared to warn him whether steps go up or down.

The deaf

Some loss of hearing affects one in three of those over 65. It appears in middle age and increases gradually. Over the age of 80 four people out of five have socially inadequate hearing. Old people are probably still too inclined to accept their hearing loss as inevitable. In fact, many could be helped by a hearing aid but less than a quarter wear them. Some need no more than the removal of the wax which has accumulated in their ears. The main trouble in old age lies in the inner ear, where the nerve cells that convert sound waves into nervous impulses degenerate, causing a perceptive type of deafness, presbycusis. The hearing loss is greatest for sounds of high frequency. As it does not at first involve the frequencies used in normal speech, it is not very disabling. Eventually, however, a stage may be reached when the old person hears only the vowels which are of low frequency and long duration, and misses consonants which are of higher frequency and shorter duration. A simple remark like 'Good morning, how are you feeling?' then sounds like 'OO— OR—IN—OW—AR—OU—EE—I?' As long as the deaf person can pick up about half of what is said, conversation is still possible but beyond that point it becomes very difficult. In struggling to fill in the missing consonants the patient may miss too much of the conversation and give answers which appear stupid. The situation will, of course, be worse if he is already mentally impaired.

Hazards of deafness

Severe deafness is a great handicap. Yet where blindness arouses sympathy, deafness, the invisible handicap, is more likely to provoke exasperation. This can cause great tensions within the family and elsewhere. Deafness also increases the danger to the patient from traffic and predisposes to road accidents. But the worst danger is isolation. To be blind cuts a person off from things. To be deaf cuts him off from people, to many a much worse hardship.

The deaf patient misinterprets what he hears. He may become paranoid, suspicious of those around him and difficult and hostile with his neighbours (see p. 244). His voice changes because he cannot hear himself speak. It then becomes harder for him to be understood as well as to understand. A further danger is that he will be thought to be mentally impaired when the real problem is that he cannot hear the questions asked. Deafness is an important reason for a misleadingly low mental score (see p. 67).

On top of all this the patient may be bearing the additional burden of tinnitus, noises generated in the inner ear. He is all too likely to give up the frustrating struggle to communicate and withdraw into a world of his own.

Conversation with the deaf

Although the deaf patient may appear to hear nothing the nurse should never talk about him as if he was not there. He may pick up just enough of the conversation to feel aggrieved and this will add to his distress. To converse with him, on the other hand, is an important way of promoting his mental well-being. When speaking with a deaf patient the nurse must be prepared to listen as well as to talk. If the patient feels that he can communicate with her, his isolation will be lessened. When she speaks to him she should speak slowly and distinctly, emphasising the consonants, but she should not shout. Some deaf patients with a symptom known as recruitment find a loud voice very distressing. The nurse should stand or sit in the patient's line of vision with her head at the same level as his and with the light on her face to facilitate lip reading. She should make sure she has caught his attention before she speaks and it may be helpful to hold his hand. She should be ready to increase her expressiveness by gesture while avoiding exaggerated grimaces.

If the patient has one ear better than the other, the nurse should use the good one. Women's voices have a higher frequency than men's, yet women often succeed in getting through to deaf patients when men fail.

Hearing aids

A deaf person can be helped if the sounds are amplified by some form of hearing aid. Powered by a small battery a hearing aid consists of a microphone, amplifier and receiver which is applied to the ear. All hearing aids, communicators and conversers have this same basic structure.

Personal hearing aids

Personal hearing aids are supplied with an individually made ear mould. Behind the ear models have now become the norm. The body worn aids still have a place however for the profoundly deaf because of their extra power and because they can be used with an ear piece to fit both ears.

Learning to use a hearing aid

The right spectacles are instantly acceptable. With hearing aids it is a different matter. It takes skill and practice to insert the ear mould, and to adjust the controls which are very small. The older patient may have stiff fingers with some loss of sensitivity.

It is also necessary for the user to accustom himself to what he hears. A person with normal hearing selects what he wants to hear. Those who live near a railway do not notice the trains. A hearing aid amplifies all sounds equally and the user has to rediscover the art of selection.

It is not therefore enough merely to give the older patient a hearing aid. He needs help and advice to make best use of it. Some hospitals have established a counselling service for this purpose.

Hearing aids in hospital

Many deaf patients admitted to a ward for the elderly will have already been supplied with an aid, but it is helpful if the nurse knows how to test whether it is in working order. A behind the ear aid is tested by turning it to maximum volume when it will emit a whistle, a condition known as feedback. The most likely reason for failure is that the battery is flat or has been put in upside down.

When talking to a hearing aid user it is best to face the patient and speak normally. To shout in his ear is counterproductive and may be very distressing.

Conversers

In the Easi-Com (Scientific & Electronic Enterprises Limited, Livingstone, West Lothian, Scotland) the receiver is large and the patient holds it to his better ear. The microphone, amplifier and battery are in a small hand held unit no bigger than a pocket torch. The apparatus is light and convenient. It has proved more acceptable than the conversers which were previously widely used. It has become an essential piece of equipment for every ward, day hospital and clinic. Even better and much cheaper is the Tandy 'Realistic' Listener with light stethoscope earpieces.

Writing

Some people are too deaf to be helped by any form of hearing aid. Those rendered totally deaf in early life may learn to lip read so well that a person talking to them is hardly aware of their handicap. Others may learn sign language. The very old, especially those with poor vision and forgetfulness as additional handicaps, are unlikely to master such techniques. For them communication in writing may be the only effective method. A pencil and writing pad should always be available. A write-on wipe-off board used with a felt tipped pen is also increasingly popular.

Deaf people at home

More can be done than is often realised to help deaf people at home. The door bell can be linked to a flashing light. The telephone can be supplied with an amplifier, loudspeaker, or a second ear piece. The telephone bell can be replaced by a light. Special fitments such as induction loops for radio and television make individual amplification less irritating to other listeners in the room. An alarm clock can be linked to a vibrating pad slipped under the pillow.

Hard of hearing clubs provide social contact. Lip reading classes may be available. The Royal National Institute for the Deaf provides information and has a range of services for the deaf of all ages including residential homes. The local social services department should know of an interpreter to help the deaf.

The deaf and blind

A few very unfortunate old people are both blind and deaf. Their problem of communication is immense, but it can be overcome to some extent. What remains is the sense of touch and this can be used to help them. Such people may be able to recognise the shape of letters traced on the palm of the hand and these can be built up into words and phrases. There is also a finger spelling alphabet which can be taught by those trained in its use. There are voluntary societies which concern themselves with this very special group. The social worker should be able to contact them.

For further reading:

BRITISH TELECOM. 1984. Help for Handicapped People.

DHSS. 1984. HA 1 (Rev) *General Guidance for Hearing Aid Users.* HMSO.

DISABLED LIVING FOUNDATION. 1979. *The Elderly Person with Failing Vision: A report to the DHSS.* HMSO.

MCCALL, R. F. 1979. *Communication Barriers in the Elderly.* Age Concern.

See also publications by the Royal National Institute for the Blind (RNIB), 224 Great Portland Street, London W1N 6AA, the Royal National Institute for the Deaf (RNID), 105 Gower Street, London WC1E 6AH, and the British Association of the Hard of Hearing, 7/11 Armstrong Road, London W3 7JL.

23
The Dying Patient

To die is as normal as to be born. Half of all deaths in the United Kingdom occur in those over the age of 75 and in the older patient there is a naturalness about death which robs it of many of its terrors. Two-thirds of all those who die will do so in hospital and the nurse who works with the elderly will become familiar with death. At least one patient in four is likely to die from the illness which brought him to hospital, and some patients are admitted specifically for terminal care. The care of the dying has special problems which involve not only the patient but also his relatives. Both require help from the whole team concerned with the patient's care.

Ways of dying

The majority of old people slip out of this life with very little pain or suffering. This is particularly evident when a previously healthy old person succumbs to an acute illness such as a coronary thrombosis, a massive cerebral haemorrhage, or an attack of pneumonia. The suffering in these cases is on the part of the relatives rather than on the part of the patient, and pneumonia has been known for generations as the old person's friend. Many old people, especially those with extensive brain damage, fade away gradually with increasing clouding of consciousness and all concerned may feel that death, when it comes, is a merciful release.

In some others, particularly those with malignant disease, and with cardiac, respiratory or renal failure, death does not come easily, but is preceded by pain, distress and disability, which may last for many weeks. Such patients often remain clear in mind to the end. They are generally younger than the average in a geriatric ward and their great need is for relief of suffering, for comfort and reassurance, and for peace of mind. Many patients come to terms with their illness eventually and exhibit a courage and serenity which comforts their family and wins the admiration of those privileged to attend them.

Reasons for going to hospital

Most people would prefer to die, as they have lived, in their own homes and among their own family, supported by their general practitioner and the community nursing team. This is not always possible, however, and more people are dying in hospital every year. The patient may live alone, or with a spouse who is herself old and frail or in a house full of small children. Because of enfeeblement, confusion or incontinence or because of the fears and anxieties of his relatives he may need more care than his family can provide

In other cases he may be transferred from another hospital or department, perhaps with his diagnosis only recently established. Or he may have come originally for treatment, perhaps with anti-mitotic drugs, but the advance of his disease may show that his need is for terminal care. Whatever the reason it is a proper function of the hospital to take care of those who are dying and there is never a time when something more cannot be done to help the patient.

Reactions of the family

Whether he leaves home or not, the patient in terminal illness remains part of his family, and they have to go through the journey together. The family has as much need of help as the patient and the staff should always be ready to listen to their anxieties.

Many people fear that death itself may be attended by great agony and distress. It is often reassuring to them to know that the end, when it comes, is likely to be quite peaceful. Most people, in fact, die in their sleep, or can be helped to do so by proper treatment. It will almost always comfort the relatives to participate as far as possible in the care of the patient and they should be given every opportunity to do so. Normally this will be by frequent visiting, but if they would like, for example, to feed the patient, the offer should be welcomed. For very ill people short visits are usually the best, but some relatives will sit quietly by the bedside for a long time and the patient may derive great comfort from their presence. Many couples come together at this time and their parting is more peaceful because of it. Children too bring their own kind of comfort to the dying and should always be made welcome. The nurse will need to be watchful, however, to see that the visitors do not exhaust either the patient or themselves.

Frequent visiting accustoms the relatives to the realities of the situation and they can see what is being done for the patient. If the patient improves a little they may feel confident enough to have him home for a time on the understanding that he can return to hospital if necessary.

Guilt feelings in the relatives

Some relatives feel guilty that the old person has had to come to hospital for his last illness, and blame themselves for failing those they love. Sometimes these guilt feelings express themselves in unjustified complaints about the patient's care or treatment. Nurses should be alert to sense this reaction on the part of the relatives and should offer them an early appointment with the social worker or the doctor. Relatives who react in this way add to their own burdens and may make the patient discontented and distrustful. Occasionally the relatives will find the situation so disturbing that they ask for the patient to be put out of his misery. They say they cannot bear to see him suffer.

Euthanasia

The deliberate ending of the patient's life, whether at his own request or that of his relatives, is known as euthanasia or mercy killing. One can have the deepest sympathy with those who feel driven to ask for this but to agree to it is to kill and to kill is morally wrong, against the law and medically unnecessary. Everything can be done to spare the patient suffering. Drugs can, of course, be given freely, and it is not necessary to take exceptional measures to prolong the patient's existence. Nothing, however, can be done with a deliberate intention of bringing the patient's life to an end. It has been well said that a doctor must not kill, but he need not prolong the act of dying. With good nursing and the careful use of drugs to relieve pain and distress it is possible to keep even the most ill patient tolerably comfortable to the last. Indeed the demand for euthanasia represents a failure in the care given to the patient and the support offered to his relatives. Where standards of care are high one seldom hears of it.

Many people fear that they will be kept alive unnecessarily when they have become helpless and a burden to others. The advocates of euthanasia make much of these anxieties, and the technical possibilities of intensive care lend substance to them. But there is a difference between being allowed to die and being killed deliberately. The Human Rights Society (27 Walpole Street, London SW3) provides a form entitled 'A Living Wish' on which a person may indicate while still in good health that while he does not desire euthanasia, he does not wish for his life to be artificially prolonged should he become helpless.

Airedale & Wharfedale
College of F.E.

Telling the patient

The question whether to tell the patient he is going to die is often discussed and there is no simple answer. Every case is different and every patient must be treated as an individual. Elderly patients who are not in immediate danger of death find it quite easy to discuss the possibility of dying and indeed sometimes pray to do so. When death is imminent, however, consciousness is often clouded so that discussion is out of the question.

At the other extreme, there is universal agreement that among those whose minds are clear, death is preceded by a perfect willingness to die. 'If I had strength enough to hold a pen', said the surgeon, William Hunter, 'I would write how pleasant and easy a thing it is to die.' People who die suddenly lose consciousness instantaneously and experience no suffering or distress at all. Even among patients with malignant disease or heart failure, who face the likelihood of a slow decline over an extended period, the problem arises less often than might be expected.

A few people seem not to wish to have their suspicions confirmed. They prefer to maintain a conspiracy of silence with their doctors and nurses. But most patients will be relieved to talk if given the opportunity. One of the objects of good care is to create an atmosphere of confidence which makes this possible. The question, 'Am I going to get better?' is better answered by another question, 'What makes you ask that?' than by an outright 'yes' or 'no'. But it is always wrong to tell a downright lie. Those who brush aside all likelihood of a fatal outcome do not succeed in comforting the patient for long. Indeed, such a response is destructive of confidence and may estrange the patient from those who care for him. As Dame Cicely Saunders put it, the real question is, 'What do you let your patients tell you?'

Many old people do not fear death so much as the act of dying and another question which is often asked is, 'How shall I die?' This is best answered by another, 'What is it that frightens you?' Dr Richard Lamerton, in his excellent book, *Care of the Dying*, gives some vivid examples of the way in which patients find their way to acceptance.

Records

It is helpful if any significant remarks made by the patient are recorded in the notes, using his actual words. It is useful also to note replies made by members of staff. In this way the whole team is made aware of the patient's changing situation.

It should surprise no one that on one day a patient will appear to accept that he is dying only to deny it the next. These are normal steps on the road to acceptance.

Mental distress

In many patients the greatest suffering arises not from pain or weakness, but from anxiety and depression. Every human being is sustained through life by the feeling that 'it can't happen to me.' When 'it' does happen the first reaction is often anger, and adjustment is difficult and painful. Moreover, some patients are troubled at this time by feelings of guilt and wonder if their present sufferings are a punishment. Most desire not to be a burden. They often feel very lonely and dying is always a venture into the unknown.

As their disease advances the truth dawns on most patients, but the staff may feel embarrassed in talking to them. A nurse who was herself dying wrote as follows: 'I know you feel insecure, don't know what to say, don't know what to do, but please believe me, if you care, you can't go wrong . . . . . All I want to know is that there will be someone to hold my hand when I need it. Death may get to be a routine to you, but it is new to me. You may not see me as unique but I have never died before. To me once is pretty unique.'

The patient is best served by a general readiness on the part of the nurse to chat with him at every opportunity about anything under the sun, so that he feels welcome and supported and loses his sense of isolation. The medical staff and the social worker will seek to give the patient the same sense of support. The doctor should be meticulous in seeking out and trying to treat any symptoms which are worrying the patient, often nothing worse than constipation. The social worker will help with any personal or domestic problems that may be causing distress. The physiotherapist may be able to relieve symptoms which do not respond to drugs. The occupational therapist may find ways to help the patient overcome his disabilities. She may also offer diversional activities so that the patient can use his time creatively and give of himself to those around him.

Spiritual help

Spiritual ministrations are of great importance at this time. While many people find in religion a resource which helps them in their dying, some religious people may be troubled by guilt or fear of what will happen to them in the after life. It is therefore part of good care to make sure that the patient has the opportunity to see the hospital chaplain or the clergyman of his choice. A clergyman may be able to help the patient find meaning in the experience through which he is passing, and, probably by listening more than talking, help him to find peace. If a person has not been active in the practice of his religion he may be reluctant to take the initiative in asking for spiritual help. But he may still be glad to accept it if it is offered. If he declines of course he should not be pressed and those who have no belief in an after life may die with as much peace and acceptance as those who do.

The hospice movement

Most of what we now know about the needs of the dying patient has been learned from the hospice movement. The first hospices were religious foundations, for example, St. Joseph's, Hackney, founded in 1883. St. Christopher's, a lay hospice founded by Dame Cicely Saunders in the 1960s pioneered the scientific as well as the humanitarian aspects of terminal care. In the past twenty years 70 hospices have been opened around the country and many more are being planned. Originally hospice care was concentrated on the patients in its beds. Now the emphasis is changing towards care in the community. Many patients stay only a short time and after relief of their symptoms return home. They may be readmitted from time to time and often for the final stages. The hospice movement now embraces outpatients, day care, rehabilitation, domiciliary care by day and night, bereavement counselling, teaching and research.

In districts where there is no hospice there may be specially trained nurses supported by the National Society for Cancer Relief and the Marie Curie Foundation. A few hospitals have pioneered a symptom control team. The team has no beds of its own but will advise on the care of dying patients in the hospital or in the community.

The principles of the hospice movement emphasise the patient's need to be fully himself in the last phase of his life. This is completely in tune with the philosophy of geriatric medicine and with good nursing care.

The control of pain

The majority of elderly patients, even those dying of cancer, do not experience severe pain. Patients with non-fatal conditions such as arthritis or post-herpetic neuralgia suffer more pain than most of those who are dying of cancer and they have to endure it for much longer. For those whose terminal illness is painful, there are many effective analgesic drugs and the most important problem is to make sure that they are given regularly, so that pain, once suppressed, need never return. The normal interval between doses is four hours but it may be less. It should not be left to the patient to say when he is in pain and to ask for relief. If the drugs are given regularly the relief of pain is self-perpetuating and the next dose is due before the effect of the last one has worn off. To be free of pain is a great help to the patient's morale, gives him confidence in those who are looking after him and leaves him free to be himself. There need be no fear of harmful drug addiction at this stage.

Simple analgesic drugs

It is not always necessary to use powerful drugs. Aspirin or paracetamol may be all that is needed. Some patients prefer compounds of aspirin or paracetamol with codeine or dextropropoxyphene, for example coproxamol (Distalgesic) or compound codeine tablets (Codis).

Morphine and diamorphine

If simple analgesics fail, most patients do best with morphine or diamorphine. Both are equally effective. About one-third of patients on these drugs experience nausea or vomiting. This can often be controlled by giving an anti-emetic drug at the same time.

Morphine and diamorphine are best given by mouth in a simple mixture with chloroform water. The usual strength is 10 mg of morphine or 5 mg of diamorphine in 5 ml of water. It is often enough to start with 2.5 ml. An advantage of the mixture is that its strength can be increased without altering the volume. The dose can be added at the bedside to 5 ml of prochlorperazine (Stemetil) syrup. After a few days, as the patient gets used to the drug, the syrup can often be withdrawn.

In hospital morphine and diamorphine are normally given four-hourly. But there are now slow release tablets of morphine, MST Continus, 10 mg, 30 mg or 60 mg, which act over 12 hours. This is convenient at home and is becoming more widely used in hospital. Morphine is also available as a suppository.

If it is necessary to give these drugs by injection, diamorphine four-hourly is preferred because it is more soluble.

Removing the cause

Sometimes the pain of terminal illness is due to a cause which can be treated directly. Bone pain from metastases responds well to non-steroid anti-inflammatory drugs (NSAID), such as indomethacin or flurbiprofen.

Pain may be due to infection and the appropriate antibiotics may help. Headache and disturbances of consciousness due to a cerebral tumour may be dramatically relieved, at least for a time, by large doses of corticosteroids, such as betamethasone or dexamethasone.

Other forms of distress

Pain is not the only problem in terminal illness. Other symptoms may be no less distressing. Old symptoms may change and new ones may develop. To control these requires constant vigilance by the caring team.

Lassitude. Lassitude, malaise and loss of appetite are common in terminal illness. They are sometimes associated with hypercalcaemia, elevation of the level of calcium in the blood. In such patients prednisolone can produce a great improvement.

Vomiting. Vomiting is often due to the drugs given to relieve pain and can be controlled by an anti-emetic such as prochlorperazine, chlorpromazine or metoclopramide. Hypercalcaemia, too, can cause vomiting which may respond to corticosteroids. Corticosteroids will also help in vomiting associated with cerebral tumours.

Patients who cannot keep down any food may be able to manage effervescent drinks. Ice cream or iced lollies may be welcomed when all other nourishment is rejected.

Dysphagia. Dysphagia, or difficulty in swallowing, may also be a problem especially when, as happens in some patients with carcinoma of the tongue or throat, it is accompanied by much pain. In such cases benzocaine lozenges or a lignocaine throat spray may be tried and the patient should have frequent mouth washes to reduce secondary infection. Some patients with carcinoma of the oesophagus can be helped surgically by the insertion of a plastic tube to maintain a passage through the growth. This may get blocked by particles of food and should be cleaned regularly by fizzy drinks or diluted hydrogen peroxide. Patients with dysphagia find it easier to swallow if they sit as upright as possible when taking nourishment. Liquidised food often helps.

Constipation. Constipation occurs in most patients who are dying and causes more misery than any other symptom. Unfortunately, the drugs which relieve pain may make it worse. When associated with faecal impaction it may provoke vomiting. A great deal of improvement may be achieved by the relief of an overloaded rectum (see Chapter 19). A laxative such as Dorbanex is usually needed routinely.

Dry mouth. A sore mouth may be due to thrush, in which case it will respond to amphotericin lozenges (Fungilin) or to nystatin suspension. A dry mouth may be caused by drugs with an atropine-like action and by dehydration. However, the giving of fluids by intravenous or nasogastric tube cannot be justified in dying patients. They can usually be kept comfortable by good mouth toilet and frequent small drinks.

Breathlessness. Breathlessness, especially in patients with heart failure, bronchitis or carcinoma of the lung may be one of the more intractable forms of distress. The correct treatment in theory is oxygen by mask but this is seldom welcomed by the patient. A wide open window may be more comforting. If there is a wheeze, salbutamol or aminophylline will probably help a little but in the end morphine and diamorphine are usually the best.

Cough. A dry cough may respond to an expectorant mixture such as Benylin or to a soothing linctus of codeine, pholcodine or diamorphine. Coughs due to growths in the larynx or throat may be soothed by frequent inhalations of menthol and benzoin or by water from a nebuliser.

A productive cough may be helped by physiotherapy to clear the bronchi and by a drug to liquify the sputum, such as bromhexine (Bisolvon). If the patient is in distress with a cough due to a respiratory infection an antibiotic may be justified.

Hiccoughs. Hiccoughs are an occasional source of distress. They often respond to the inhalation of 7 per cent carbon dioxide. If this is not available the level of CO_2 in the blood can be raised quickly by getting the patient to breathe for a few moments in and out of a paper bag. Where hiccough persists a phenothiazine tranquilliser or metoclopramide may be effective.

Fungating ulcers. Fungating ulcers, usually in the breast, may cause much distress and smell if not kept clean. Dressings of eusol and paraffin have been superseded by liquid paraffin mixed with 4 per cent povidone iodine solution (Betadine) in a ratio of 4 to 1. The mixture is used to clean the wound and then gauze soaked in it is applied as a dressing. A drop of Nilodor on the dressing and an Airwick or scented air freshener is often useful also.

The death bed

Unless he has asked to be moved to a single room it is generally better for the patient to die in the general ward and not to be separated from his companions at the end. He is less likely to be lonely. The others may be reassured to observe that the dying person is treated with loving care and that death, when it comes, is peaceful and unalarming. Only if the dying patient is distressed and noisy and cannot be made comfortable by medical treatment and good nursing, is it necessary to move him to a side ward.

In his last hours the patient may be more comfortable if he is propped up with his head well supported rather than lying flat. If he appears restless he should be moved gently and often. If he is aware of his surroundings he is likely to feel a need for light and air. Above all he must know that he is not alone. In hospices for the dying it is a rule that no one should die without someone sitting by his bed. With present staffing in hospital it can seldom be a nurse, but it is an important contribution which the relatives can make to the dying patient, provided that the staff look in frequently to offer support and encouragement. The patient may sweat profusely while he is dying and may need to be sponged. He should not be allowed to suffer thirst and regular mouth toilet is important to the end. The death rattle occurs when the patient is too weak to cough up secretions in his trachea. Provided the patient is unconscious the distress which this noise causes to others can be eased by laying the patient on his side and raising the foot of the bed so that the secretions drain into his mouth. An injection of atropine to dry the mucous membranes may also be helpful at this stage.

After the death

After death has occurred the relatives, when they are ready, should be gently led aside. It may help them to talk about the person who has just left them, but they may feel stunned and unable to take in what has happened. Before they leave the ward the nurse should make sure that they receive clear instructions about the death certificate and other formalities. This normally means a visit to the hospital to see the administrator on the day following death.

The nurse's reaction

When the relatives have gone the nurse still has to wash and lay out the body, a last act of service which she will perform with all possible gentleness and respect. The nurse herself may grieve when a well loved patient dies and she may need to discuss her feelings with other members of the team. Such emotions are entirely natural and the more the staff are seen to care, the more the relatives and other patients will be comforted. Death, though it causes grief to those who are bereaved, is a necessity in the economy of nature and, many believe, is the way by which the person who has died enters a fuller life and realises the meaning of his existence.

Reaction in the ward

In many hospitals it is customary to draw the bed curtains when the dead body is removed, not to speak afterwards of the one who has died, to pretend that nothing has happened. It is far better, particularly in longer stay wards, for the staff to be ready to talk with the other patients about the person who has gone. In this way all can express their feelings and come to terms with reality.

For further reading:

HECTOR, W. & WHITFIELD, S. 1982. *Nursing Care of the Dying Patient and the Family*. London: Heinemann.

KUBLER ROSS, E. 1981. *Living with Death and Dying*. London: Souvenir Press.

LAMERTON, R. 1980. *Care of the Dying*. London: Penguin.

SMITH, C. R. 1982. *Social Work with the Dying and the Bereaved*. British Association of Social Workers.

TWYCROSS, R. G. & LACK, S. 1984. *Therapeutics in Terminal Cancer*. London: Pitman.

24
Nurse Staffing and Standards of Care

The standards of nursing care advocated in this book cannot be achieved without sufficient staff. In the National Health Service there is a constant tension between the demands of the work and the resources, both human and financial, available to maintain good care. As the cuts bite and financial stringency increases, the problem is often how to make the best use of the limited resources available. This may mean closing beds in order to maintain proper staff patient ratios. It is always better to have fewer beds well staffed than more beds poorly staffed. Understaffing inevitably leads to lower standards, neglect of patients, poor morale, justified complaints and ultimately scandal.

The changing scene

In recent years work in geriatric wards has become increasingly acute. In 1972 the average length of stay in a geriatric ward in Great Britain was 105 days. In Hastings in 1983 the figure was 36 days.

Figures for the average length of stay are disproportionately influenced by long-stay patients and a more telling figure is the median length of stay, the time by which half of all patients have been discharged. In England and Wales in 1980 the median length of stay in geriatric wards was 20 days. In Hastings in 1982 it was 12 days. The comparable figure for an acute medical ward taking patients of all ages was 7 days.

High turnover, though stimulating, makes increased demands upon the nurse. More new patients with acute illness mean more effort, more investigation, more paper work, more deaths. Amidst all this acute work the nurse must try to create an atmosphere of rehabilitation and provide longer term care for very dependent patients. For all these reasons geriatric wards need more staff than general medical and surgical wards, but they seldom get them.

Wholetime equivalents

One wholetime nurse works 37.5 hours a week. This is counted as one wholetime equivalent (WTE). The hours of part-time nurses are added together and, when they total 37.5, this counts as 1 WTE. Thus, two nurses, one working 20 hours and the other 17.5, would make 1 WTE. Staff ratios are expressed as 1 WTE to so many patients.

Staffing guidelines

There are no official standards which must be observed and guidelines promulgated by the DHSS in 1974 have been withdrawn. The best guidelines are those of the British Geriatrics Society which recommends a nurse patient ratio of 1 to 1.16. This provides 20.7 WTE to cover a ward of 24 beds round the clock.

In practice funds are seldom available to provide staff up to this standard. Usually wards are staffed to about 80 per cent of BGS standards, approximately 1 WTE to 1.5 beds. This normally allows four staff to be on duty during the day, three in the evening and two at night for a ward of 24 beds. It is recommended that 40 per cent of ward staff should be trained, 30 per cent in training and 30 per cent untrained. Where there are fewer nurses in training there should be a higher proportion of trained staff. In non-training wards 50 per cent of the staff should be trained.

These staffing levels are marginally better than those recommended for general medical and surgical wards where the degree of patient dependency is usually less. They are based on the assumption that the nurse will be relieved of all non-nursing duties.

Housekeeping teams

Nurses can concentrate better on patient care if a ward housekeeping team relieves them of non-nursing duties. This includes making beds when not occupied by patients, cleaning lockers, supervising patients' property, serving meals and preparing light refreshments. The ward clerk may be a member of the housekeeping team with responsibility for the reception of visitors, answering the telephone, running messages and maintaining the medical notes in good order. The team also maintains ward supplies of linen, provisions, stationery and containers for laboratory specimens. It may operate the ward launderette.

The housekeeping team can be a great help to the nurses but it is vital that they work closely together.

Communication within the team

All members of the team should have the same objectives and the same understanding of what they are trying to achieve for each patient. Moreover nurses and auxiliaries who bear the brunt of day-to-day patient care with all its anxieties, should feel supported from above. This is achieved by good communication, not only within the ward but within the unit as a whole and within the hospital of which the unit forms a part. At ward level the doctor's rounds are a crucial part of this process. In a geriatric ward the doctor, the nurse and the patient treat each other as equals. A round should include discussion with each patient about his progress and the aims of his treatment.

Not all nurses can attend every ward round and the nurse in charge will keep her team in close touch with what is going on by daily discussion. The nursing process is invaluable to this end (see p. 69).

The housekeeper must be kept in the picture, for her staff bring their own brand of reassurance to the patient. In addition every week should see at least one ward meeting between the nurses and the remedial therapists. This should, if possible, also be attended by a doctor and a social worker. The clinical teacher should come with the learners. There will also be regular meetings between the sisters and charge nurses and the nurse manager. It is an advantage if these too can be attended by the medical, administrative and remedial staff from time to time. The good nurse manager should not only be an expert in the technicalities of nursing the elderly but should have a close personal understanding of all her nurses and be ready to counsel and support them. This kind of activity creates a good atmosphere and high morale. These points are developed in another book in the Modern Nursing Series, *Leadership and the Nurse*, by Margaret Schurr (this book is out of print and should be found in nursing libraries).

Quality of care

High standards of care cannot be achieved without sufficient staff. Attention must also be given to the quality of care given by each member of staff. In an effort to achieve this the Doncaster Group of Hospitals has a system of Nursing Care Audits. These provide a check-list against which nurses of all grades can assess the standards of their unit and their own attitudes and performance.

Extracts from a Nursing Care Audit
General:
Do the practices and procedures adopted seek to assist the elderly person to function at full mental and physical potential and preserve his individuality?

Assessment and rehabilitation:

Is there a satisfactory system which enables you to assess accurately the physical and psychological needs of newly admitted patients?

Are programmes of care and rehabilitation based on medical, nursing, functional and social assessment? How often are they reviewed?

Are you conversant with the rehabilitation programme arranged jointly by the occupational therapist, the physiotherapist and the speech therapist? Are these programmes continued in their absence?

When assisting patients to practise a skill, do you first gain their confidence, promote a friendly optimistic atmosphere at all times, and encourage the patients to help themselves?

Individuality:

Do you consider the personal preferences of the patients when you arrange the following?

    (a) Time for getting up
    (b) Selection of clothes to be worn
    (c) Activities to be pursued
    (d) Spending personal monies
    (e) Receiving visitors
    (f) Refreshment
    (g) Bathing times
    (h) Bedtime

Are the patients encouraged to have their personal belongings around them?

Do you recognise that the patient has a right to privacy and solitude if he wishes?

Personal appearance and dress:

Are your patients encouraged and helped to take an interest and pride in their personal appearance?

Are the following requirements met?

    (a) The hair is tidy and appropriately styled
    (b) Hearing aids are available and in working order
    (c) Spectacles are available and regularly cleaned
    (d) Dentures are worn and clearly marked
    (e) Facial hair is removed if desired
    (f) Suitable underclothes are worn
    (g) Trousers are well fitting and correctly fastened
    (h) The ward has a supply of belts and braces
    (i) Shoes are worn unless contra-indicated

Are long mirrors strategically placed in the ward to encourage patients to take a pride in their appearance?

Is every effort made to ensure that the clothes worn by disabled patients are of suitable design?

Are dressing aids available on the ward for those patients who have been assessed as needing them?
  (a) Stocking aid
  (b) Long-handled shoehorn
  (c) Elastic shoe laces
  (d) Dressing stick

Are you conversant with the correct use of these aids?

When helping patients to dress do you ensure that their clothes are put out for them in order?

Communicating with the patient:

Do you always address the patient in the correct manner and treat him with dignity and respect?

Do you ensure that all nursing treatments and procedures are fully explained to the patient before they are carried out and that privacy is afforded to him at all times?

Are you aware that a calm and friendly ward atmosphere is of therapeutic value to the patient? Do you try to promote this at all times?

Is every opportunity taken to establish a good rapport with patients irrespective of their response, attractiveness and personality?

Are you encouraged to sit and converse with and listen to the patient?

Is the day room seating arranged in a manner conducive to easy communication between patients?

The deaf and blind:

Is every effort made to keep deaf and blind patients aware of their surroundings and to ensure that they are introduced to all new members of staff?

Are you aware of the correct way to address a deaf patient and of the need to speak slowly and distinctly?

Are blind patients always spoken to when approached and made aware of the reason for your presence?

Mental impairment and restlessness:

Are you aware of the functional limitations of the mentally impaired patient? Do you understand the need for established daily routines and purposeful activities?

Are you aware that restlessness and confusion need to be investigated in order to establish the cause and to ensure that the appropriate treatment is given?

What advice has been given to you about the use of safety sides?

Bladder and bowel:

Are you aware of the importance of observing and recording accurately the details of the pattern of the patient's bladder and bowel function?

The seriously ill patient:

Is every effort made to meet the needs of the seriously ill patient when planning the work of the ward?

Are you conversant with the agreed procedures for the prevention and treatment of pressure sores?

Relatives:

Are relatives encouraged to participate in the care and rehabilitation of the patient if they so wish?

Do relatives receive guidance on the management of the patient at home and instructions in the use of nursing aids and equipment?

Are bereaved relatives treated with particular consideration, sympathy and understanding?

Research:

Do you appreciate the value of research and its contribution to improved patient care?

Are you encouraged to participate in new projects?

For further reading:

BRITISH GERIATRICS SOCIETY AND ROYAL COLLEGE OF NURSING. 1974. *Improving Geriatric Care in Hospital*. Royal College of Nursing.

RHYS HEARN, C. 1979. Staffing Geriatric Wards, *Nursing Times* Occasional Paper 11. *Nursing Times*, **75** (17): 45−52.

RHYS HEARN, C. 1981. Experience with the Rhys Hearn geriatric workload package, *Nursing Times* Occasional Paper 12. *Nursing Times*, **77** (3): 9−12.

Appendix

The following is a leaflet issued by Hastings Health Authority as information for visitors:

Hastings Health Authority

Departments of Medicine and Mental Health for the Elderly

St. Helen's Hospital	Tel. Hastings 427090
Bexhill Hospital	Tel. Bexhill 212121
Battle Hospital	Tel. Battle 2030
Eversfield Hospital	Tel. Hastings 436351
Hellingly Hospital	Tel. Hailsham 844391

Information for Visitors

Consultant Physicians:

Dr. R. E. Irvine

Dr. T. M. Strouthidis

Consultant Psychiatrist:

Dr. T. Venkateswarlu

Nursing Officers:

St. Helen's	Mrs. M. E. Couchman
Bexhill & Eversfield	Miss S. B. Ward
Battle	Mr. G. Anderson
Mental Health	Mr. B. A. Williams

The Departments

The Departments of Medicine for the Elderly and Mental Health for the Elderly are primarily concerned to provide a service for patients aged 76 and over. All are under the care of a consultant.

The Departments have units at St. Helen's, Bexhill, Battle, Eversfield and Hellingly Hospitals. We all work closely together. We are concerned to provide an appropriate environment for each stage of the patients' treatment. For most this will involve at some time a move from one ward or unit to another.

Patients are admitted as soon as their doctor requests it and most go home when they are better. For those who will not get better we aim to offer care, comfort and support.

St. Helen's Hospital

St. Helen's has facilities for the investigation and treatment of acute illness. It takes patients from the whole District of the Hastings Health Authority. New patients normally come to Wards 4, 4a, 5, 5a and a few to 3a. Ward 9 is for rehabilitation and preparation for home. Wards 11 and 12 offer slow stream rehabilitation and continuing care for the most disabled and dependent patients. St. Helen's Day Hospital provides rehabilitation and treatment for patients after they leave hospital, and for a few while they are in the wards.

Ward 3a is primarily for medical treatment and rehabilitation of patients transferred from the orthopaedic wards at the Royal East Sussex Hospital.

Bexhill Unit

The Bexhill Unit provides rehabilitation and a day hospital, primarily for Bexhill residents. Patients normally move to Bexhill after a period of treatment at St. Helen's. They take part with the day patients in a full programme of activities which lasts until the afternoon. The Bexhill Unit is not large enough to meet all needs. To help as many local residents as possible, it may be necessary for some patients to move elsewhere after a period of treatment.

Battle Hospital

Battle Hospital provides continuing care for those who live in the vicinity. In the summer it also takes holiday admissions. It has more beds than are needed for Battle residents and takes some patients from Bexhill and Hastings. Every effort is made to select those for whom this will not prove a hardship. A few patients are taken for day care.

Eversfield Hospital

Eversfield Hospital provides continuing care and holiday admissions for those in the vicinity. Eversfield has a patient/relative Association. This aims to express the consumer's view of our service and to make suggestions for improvement. Ask the staff how you can join in its meetings.

Both Eversfield and Battle Hospital provide a programme of activities and outings. Patients are free to take part or not as they wish.

Department of Mental Health for the Elderly

The principal aim of the Department is to help its patients to remain at home as long as possible.

The consultant psychiatrist heads a professional team including a psychologist, community psychiatric nurses, occupational therapy staff, social workers and volunteers.

The Department has an assessment unit in Ward 3 at St. Helen's and beds at Hellingly Hospital. Patients are admitted to either hospital and some come to St. Helen's for day care.

All patients have an initial assessment, usually in their own home, by a member of the team and some then come to hospital. Most go home when they are better. For those who do not get better we try to offer an alternative form of care.

Visitors

Your visits make an important contribution to the patient's treatment. We are concerned that all patients should maintain contact with their family and friends. You are welcome to visit any time between 9 a.m. and 9 p.m. Please bring children with you if you wish.

Patients who are ill tire easily and it is usually best to visit frequently but for short periods. Even when the patient seems unaware of your presence, it will probably be helpful to him and to you to spend time just sitting at the bedside.

Convalescent patients may appreciate longer visits but an hour is usually enough. You will appreciate that activities relating to the patient's treatment and rehabilitation take place throughout the day and the person you wish to see may not be immediately available. Please introduce yourself at every visit to the nurse in charge of the ward. Every effort will be made to help you and to keep you informed.

You are welcome to participate in the patient's care and the nurses will be happy to discuss with you how you may do this. If you can take the patient for an outing or are able to have him home from time to time it will do much to sustain his morale.

We need you to tell us about the patient as a person. The more you can tell us about him and his likes and dislikes, the better we shall understand him.

Overnight Stay

If you have to stay overnight because your relative is very ill, the hospital can provide you with a place to rest. The nurse in charge will make the necessary arrangements.

Clothing

Elderly people in hospital are usually better for being up and dressed in their own clothes and walking shoes. These should be clearly marked with the patient's name. Towels and night clothes will be provided by the hospital if necessary.

Your help in keeping the patient supplied with regular changes of clothing will be appreciated. Please take suitcases home. We have no room for them in our overcrowded wards.

Laundry

The hospital laundry is not designed to process patient's personal laundry on a regular basis but it will endeavour to cope with emergencies when alternative personal arrangements cannot be made. Eversfield and Bexhill have launderettes, but these are not available at St. Helen's or Battle. Clothes for washing will be left in a bag on the bedside locker for you to collect. Your help in keeping the patients neatly dressed will help their recovery. It is most helpful for all patients' clothing to be marked with their name.

Property and Valuables

All items of value, including glasses, dentures and money are checked and listed on admission. If further items of value, particularly rings, are brought in or removed after the patient has been admitted, **it is important to tell the staff**. The hospital cannot be responsible for valuables unless handed in for safe keeping and an official receipt obtained. Money will be banked and returned by cheque. If cash in excess of £10 is required, 48 hours notice is required. There may be difficulties at the weekend.

You can help by ensuring that the patient has regular small amounts of money for newspapers, toilet articles and other goods from the hospital shop or trolley.

Social Work Staff

If there are difficulties about the patient's personal affairs or his return home, please make an early appointment to see the social workers at St. Helen's and Bexhill who are available to help you on every weekday. There is a solution to most problems, even in old age, and they will help you to find it.

Medical Staff

The doctors are always glad to see you, particularly during ward rounds, but also by appointment. The nurse in charge will help you. At Bexhill the doctors are Dr. P. M. Kendall and Dr. M. Evans. At Battle, Dr. D. G. C. Griffith and Dr. P. Mogan. At Eversfield, Dr. S. C. Paget and Dr. I. M. G. Torkington.

Chaplain

The Church of England Chaplain to all the hospitals is the Rev. David Godwin. He visits the wards regularly and is always available if you want to see him. The nurse in charge of the ward can contact him on your behalf.

Services are held regularly in all the hospitals.

The Chapel at St. Helen's is always open and you are very welcome to use it. It is off the corridor between Wards 4 and 2.

There is a service every Sunday at 9.30 a.m. Holy Communion is brought to the wards regularly.

Your own Priest, Minister or Rabbi is, of course, welcome to visit at any time.

Telephone Enquiries

Except in emergencies it is best if telephone enquires can be made between 9 a.m. and 5 p.m. when a ward clerk is available to answer the telephone. It is helpful also if one of a family or group of friends can make the telephone enquiries and then inform the others.

Mobile Telephones (payfones)

These can usually be brought to the patients' bedside (provided they are able to use them) for direct personal contact with friends and relatives. These and other payfones situated throughout the hospital may be used by relatives and visitors for outgoing calls only.

Medicines

It is most helpful if you can bring in all the medicines which the patient has been taking at home and any treatment card issued by the family doctor.

Transport

There is a bus service to each hospital but the timetables change. We suggest you telephone the headquarters of the local bus company on Hastings 431770. British Rail enquiries on Hastings 429325.

Questions and Suggestions

If you have any questions to ask or suggestions to make, please feel free to talk to the staff. If you prefer to write, there is a suggestion box on every ward.

Index